REENVISIONING THERAPY WITH WOMEN OF COLOR
A BLACK FEMINIST HEALING PERSPECTIVE

LANI V. JONES

NASW PRESS

National Association of Social Workers
Washington, DC

Kathryn Conley Wehrmann, PhD, LCSW, *President*
Angelo McClain, PhD, LICSW, *Chief Executive Officer*

Cheryl Y. Bradley, *Publisher*
Rachel Meyers, *Acquisitions Editor*
Julie Gutin, *Managing Editor*
Sarah Lowman, *Project Manager*
Kathleen P. Baker, *Copyeditor*
Juanita Doswell, *Proofreader*
Matthew White, *Indexer*

Cover by Britt Engen, Metadog Design Group
Interior design, composition, and eBook conversions by Xcel Graphic Services
Printed and bound by Integrated Books International

First impression: April 2020

© 2020 by the NASW Press

All rights reserved. No part of this book may be reproduced or transmitted in any form or by any means, electronic or mechanical, including photocopying, recording, or by any information storage and retrieval system, without permission in writing from the publisher.

Library of Congress Cataloging-in-Publication Data

Names: Jones, Lani V. (Lani Valencia), author.
Title: Reenvisioning therapy with women of color : a Black feminist healing perspective / Lani V. Jones.
Description: Washington, DC : NASW Press, [2020] | Includes bibliographical references and index. | Summary: "This book explores the complex mental health experiences of Women of Color. The book, a primer for therapists and educators, will help mental health therapists gain a deeper understanding of the complex and multiplicative problems that Women of Color bring into treatment, assist therapists in developing culturally responsive intervention skills, and present key elements critical to Black feminist therapeutic philosophy, theory, and practice"—Provided by publisher.
Identifiers: LCCN 2019057029 (print) | LCCN 2019057030 (ebook) | ISBN 9780871015525 (paperback) | ISBN 9780871015532 (ebook)
Subjects: LCSH: African American women—Mental health. | African American Women—Psychology. | Feminist therapy.
Classification: LCC RC451.4.M58 J66 2020 (print) | LCC RC451.4.M58 (ebook) | DDC 616.890082—dc23
LC record available at https://lccn.loc.gov/2019057029
LC ebook record available at https://lccn.loc.gov/2019057030

Printed in the United States of America

Down-Home Philosophy

By Francine Guy, Woman of Color, consumer–survivor

Sometimes
you just have to surrender
cause it's outa yo' hands
And say—hey—let it be
Cause it's outa yo' hands
Sometimes.
Mama told me 'bout it
granddaddy preached about it
some of us still wrestling with it.
Sometimes
You just have to watch and wait
Cause it aint yours to control
And you done all you can anyway
And it aint yo' move no way.
Sometimes—
But when the watchin' and waitin'
And weighin' is done
You gotta be ready
to move.

Contents

Preface vii

Acknowledgments ix

Introduction 1

Chapter 1: Women of Color's Mental Health Matters: *Mujeres de Color, en la Lucha* (Women of Color, in the Struggle) 13

Chapter 2: Developing a Black Feminist Analysis for Mental Health Practice: From Theory to Praxis 23

Chapter 3: Culturally Responsive Services 43

Chapter 4: Understanding Power and Powerlessness in Therapy with Women of Color 55

Chapter 5: Applying Black Feminist Therapy Approaches to Women of Color in Therapy 67

Chapter 6: Case Illustrations 81

Chapter 7: Claiming Your Connections: An Evidence-Based Psychosocial Competence Group Intervention Grounded in Black Feminism 95

Chapter 8: Conclusion: Black Feminist Therapy, a 21st Century Imperative 113

Appendix: Terminology 119

References 123

Index 143

About the Author 149

Preface

Whether Women of Color are dealing with disrespect, denigration, microaggressions, or violence or trying to survive in the current volatile sociopolitical climate, our emotional wellness is compromised. We are constantly expected to shoulder the weight of others physically, psychologically, spiritually, and even financially, with no attention to self, and our emotional labor is constantly demanded. No matter how many times we are praised for being strong and sassy, chances are that the psychosocial pressures of racism, patriarchy, and misogyny are taking a negative toll on our mental health. This has been true for quite some time. We are emotionally exhausted, and as a consequence, our mental health is at risk. We need person-centered, politically informed perspectives that position therapy within a cultural context, privileging race, gender, and all other "isms."

From this position, therapeutic perspectives, such as Black feminist therapy, empower Woman of Color to potentially address aspects of emotional and social transformation, nurture self, and make meaning of her multiple identities. Through these actions, therapists can eliminate or reduce those psychosocial stressors that often lead to severe and persistent mental health distress and disorders among Women of Color.

With this in mind, I set out to write an unapologetic book about Women of Color and their mental health, illness, and wellness. I was thrilled to write this book because although I am exhausted by my own professional and familial psychological wounds, I am inspired by the healing possibilities of Black feminist therapy. I am also excited to help dispel the myths about why Women of Color do not need or seek mental health treatment and to show that Women of Color have been here the whole time, pleading for culturally responsive treatment. Over the course of my 25-plus years as a therapist, I have always wanted to read a book about the complex but vivid mental health and wellness experiences of Women of Color, by a Woman of Color. That book did not exist, so I set out to write it.

Women of Color can no longer afford to be silent or go unheard. We must tell the world, and each other, about our struggles with mental health issues, as well as our disappointment with mental health systems in the United States. The authority and privilege to write this book has been offered to me by other Black feminists (as well as consumers) who handed this challenge to me. As a focus group participant shared,

> We're framing all this stuff and then we're going to hand it to . . . our community of Black feminist scholars to operationalize. . . . Because I think this [Black feminist therapy] is what we need as Women of Color, what our communities need. . . . Sometimes you have to write the book you need to read. And I think that's really what this is all about. . . . What are the tools? What's the awareness that we need? And how can Lani be one of many people [who] come together to help us shape that?

I view this book as a blueprint for therapists and educators, as well as a self-help book for all women. My intention in writing this book is to help mental health therapists gain a deeper understanding of the complex and multiplicative problems that Women of Color bring into treatment, assist therapists in developing foundational culturally responsive intervention skills, and present key elements and proficiencies critical to Black feminist therapy. Specifically, I crystallize the origins of Black feminist theories and perspectives, explore the current patterns of mental health utilization and service needs among Women of Color, and detail foundational strategies for using Black feminist perspectives in mental health treatment. Black feminist therapy is an arena in which I establish myself as a comrade to Communities of Color. I do not pretend to know everything about the experiences of Women of Color who engage in or seek mental health therapy; however, through this book, I share my knowledge and experiences and the expertise of other Women of Color so that I can assist therapists in reaching their goals to radically transform therapeutic practices. Hence, my thoughts are not the definitive take on Women of Color's mental health needs and Black feminist therapy.

My courage to write, fight, educate, struggle, and strive in the field of mental health and in the academy comes from the many Women of Color who stood before me. They taught me that our stories, like our lives, are complex and multiplicative, beautiful, hopeful, and often disregarded. I hope to honor their lives, commitment, and dedication.

Acknowledgments

Much of what I have learned over the years as a Black feminist scholar-practitioner came as the result of my work with Women of Color consumers, all of whom inspired me and subconsciously contributed a tremendous amount to the content of this book through their stories of pain, fear, hope, joy, and success. I am grateful to have been invited into their healing circle.

I am overwhelmed in all humbleness and gratefulness to all those who have helped me conceptualize and operationalize my Black feminist therapy ideas, well above the level of simplicity and into something concrete. A deep gratitude of thanks to my Sista therapists' comrades, Vanessa Jackson, Kendra C. Roberson, Deborah R. Brome, Francine L. Guy, and Michelle A. Harris who served as my Black feminist therapy "Think Tank." Your love, dreams, prayers, and Black girl magic gave me the confidence to persevere. To my fierce feminist-Sista friend, Beverly Guy-Sheftall, your critical inquiry, dynamism, vision, candor, and care deeply inspired me to carry out this project. This book is built on your Black feminist legacy.

I would like to say thanks to my colleagues for their constant encouragement. I extend a special thanks to Lynn A. Warner for your friendship and support. You have stood by me through my every struggle and all my success. Many thanks to my graduate students Nelia M. Quezada, Lauren Cestone, and Nadine George for your support during my research and writing. Y'all were my eyes when my vision failed me, my strength when I was depleted. I appreciate you!

I am extremely grateful to my family because my hopes and dreams are your hopes and dreams. Grandmother, Ethel May Jones Batts, a Black feminist warrior of your time, your spirit carried me to the end. My sister, Melanie C. M. Jones, your love, prayers, and sacrifice sustain me. Maya I. Campbell, I write this for you Goddaughter; may this be a healing tool for you and your generation.

To NASW Press staff members Cheryl Y. Bradley, Rachel Meyers, Stella Donovan, and Sarah Lowman, thank you for your support from start to finish. I am grateful. To my Brother Angelo McClain, your leadership at NASW is a testimony to our work in delivering the best possible care in social work.

To my little sisters of DST, Inc., Sorors Nathaalie M. Carey and Dorcey Applyrs, thank you for always showing up big: Big in vision, Big in protest, and Big in love.

Asè

Introduction

*I am the first and the last. I am the honored one and the scorned one.
I am the whore and the holy one. I am the wife and the virgin. I am the
barren one and many are my daughters. I am the silence that you cannot
understand. I am the utterance of my name.*

—Julie Dash (2006, p. 92), from an ancient gnostic verse,
"The Thunder, Perfect Mind" (see Gnostic Society Library, n.d.)

Since 2006, social media feeds have been flooded with the hashtag #MeToo, a campaign founded by African American social activist Tarana Burke to help survivors of sexual violence realize they are not alone. #MeToo was further ignited by actress Alyssa Milano in 2017 with the tweet, "If you've been sexually harassed or assaulted write 'me too' as a reply to this tweet," and it quickly turned into a movement. In a show of solidarity, many women—and some men—have shared their experiences of sexual assault, rape, harassment, and other forms of sexual abuse.

The onslaught of divulgences led me to ask the questions "What if there was a #MeToo mental health movement for Women of Color with mental illness and emotional distress? And how would America represent this hashtag for Women of Color?" These questions moved me to exhale (ahhh), not forgetting to BREATHE (balance, reflection, energy, association, transparency, healing, empowerment), as so eloquently constructed by my colleagues Evans, Bell, and Burton (2017) in *Black Women's Mental Health: Balancing Strength and Vulnerability*. The BREATHE model highlights processes that encourage Women of Color to practice mental health wellness.

Conversely, Women of Color know that our mental health suffers when we are not able to BREATHE through the brunt of racism, sexism, other forms of oppression, and the daily pressures of familial and societal responsibility. In the United States, approximately 7.5 million Women of Color have a diagnosed mental health disorder, and as many as 7.5 million more may be similarly affected but not have been diagnosed (K. Davis, 2005). In addition, Women of Color experience substantial individual, interpersonal, and socioeconomic stressors at a higher rate than do their White counterparts (Alegría et al., 2002; L. C. Jackson & Greene, 2000). Compared with their White peers, Women of Color are more likely to be single parents, be overworked and underpaid, possess fewer financial resources, live in impoverished communities, and experience intimate partner and community violence (DeNavas-Walt, Proctor, & Smith, 2008; McKinnon, 2003). Moreover, Women of Color experience substantial barriers to receiving mental health and substance abuse services, and the services they do receive often lack cultural and ethnic awareness (Borum, 2012; T. A. Davis & Ancis, 2012; Institute of Medicine, Committee on Understanding and Eliminating Racial and Ethnic Disparities in Health Care, 2003). These are the oppressive psychological and social realities faced by many Women of Color in the United States.

As a Black feminist therapist–scholar, I have prioritized my commitment to the psychosocial wellness of Women of Color in our struggle for liberation. I understand our collective pain, rage, sadness, and loneliness, along with our brilliance, determination, collective experience, creativity, power, and sisterhood. I have worked thoughtfully to develop culturally relevant therapeutic strategies and interventions to assist in healing our minds, souls, and physical selves. I use Black feminist therapy to help women cope with, and resolve, work and family problems, negative behavioral patterns, conflicting beliefs and feelings, and related physical symptoms. I have come to see the therapeutic process as an approach through which to view, understand, acknowledge, and intervene without judgment and through which to engage in informed, explicit discussions about women's life stories and how they survive and thrive as Women of Color. In addition, I offer my whole self in the therapeutic process, acknowledging my privileges and struggles and recognizing my intersecting oppressions.

To facilitate this journey toward the utilization of culturally relevant therapeutic perspectives, I challenge the homogeneous (that is, White, middle class, male), hierarchical, and dualistic limitations of traditional feminist therapy to be more inclusive of race, class, and sexual orientation in the development and utilization of Black feminist perspectives (Boyd-Franklin, 1991; Greene, 1997; L. C. Jackson & Greene, 2000; C. B. Williams, 2000). Such a culturally relevant feminist model of understanding and treating mental health issues addresses all forms of marginalization and discrimination simultaneously rather than privileging gender issues alone. This process of cultural relevance involves enhancing the understanding of Women of Color in context, developing a power-balanced relationship with them, and adapting a healing approach geared to the client's needs. Therapists adopting such a perspective are not required to abandon their theoretical and practice approaches to therapy but rather to adopt a lens through which to better understand, acknowledge, and intervene that is based on the client's life experiences in a cultural, ethnic, and economic context while simultaneously integrating diverse and pluralistic healing approaches into techniques and interventions.

DEFINING WOMEN OF COLOR

Although the term "Women of Color" is used to represent various cultural and ethnic groups of women, I use the term throughout this book to represent women in the United States who are of the African diaspora—some of whom may consider themselves Black and others who may consider themselves Latina—whose shared experiences of marginalization and oppression can lead to negative social, economic, and psychological consequences. This term is used in solidarity with women of African, African American, Caribbean (West Indian), Indigenous, and Latin descent as a commitment to develop interventions and processes specific to their context. To be clear, this definition of Women of Color does not include women of European or Asian descent.

I also believe that it is important for me to provide a brief commentary about my choice to capitalize and not capitalize adjectives or words that refer to women's identities (for example, White, Black, Women of Color). In general, I follow the lead of previous contributors to Black feminist theory and feminist therapy. For example, many influential Black scholars and Black feminist authors have capitalized "Black" because it refers to a specific form of theory and identity within feminisms. Thus, I chose to capitalize all references to specific identities such as Black, White, Latin, and Women of Color.

Language is an essential element in understanding the psychosocial, economic, and political struggle of most non-White women in the United States. Shifts in the words we use to describe each other and groups of people (that is, "others") often reflect our collective progress toward a world in which all women feel respected and included. Ethnicity is a neglected dimension of the heterogeneity among people of African and Latin descent (D. R. Williams et al., 2007). Although there are important commonalities in the experiences of persons of African and Latin descent, there is also ethnic variation within this population. Approximately 6 percent of the U.S. Black population is foreign born, and 10 percent of the Black population (3.4 million) is of foreign parentage (U.S. Census Bureau, 2010). There are more Black and Latino immigrants in the United States than there are Indian, Chinese, or Japanese immigrants (Barnes & Bennett, 2002; Grieco & Cassidy, 2001; Guzmán, 2001). In fact, Latinos and Blacks from the Caribbean constitute the largest subgroup of U.S. immigrants of persons of African descent (D. R. Williams et al., 2007).

The term "Women of Color" surfaced in the late 1970s to encompass all women experiencing multiple layers of oppression with race and ethnicity as a commonality. As explained by Loretta Ross,

> Y'all know where the term "women of color" came from? Who can say that? See, we're bad at transmitting history. In 1977, a group of Black women from Washington, DC, went to the National Women's Conference, that [former President] Jimmy Carter gave $5 million to have as part of the World Decade for Women. There was a conference in Houston, TX. This group of Black women carried into that conference something called "The Black Women's Agenda" because the organizers of the conference—Bella Abzug, Ellie Smeal, and what have you—had put together a three-page "Minority Women's Plank" in a 200-page document that these Black women thought was somewhat inadequate. (Giggles in background) So they actually formed a group called Black Women's Agenda to come [sic] to Houston with a Black women's plan of action that they wanted the delegates to vote to substitute for the "Minority Women's Plank" that was in the proposed plan of action. Well, a funny thing happened in Houston: when they took the Black Women's Agenda to Houston, then all the rest of the "minority" women of color wanted to be included in the "Black Women's Agenda." Okay? Well, [the Black women] agreed . . . but you could no longer call it the "Black Women's Agenda." And it was in those negotiations in Houston [that] the term "women of color" was created. (as cited in Wade, 2011, para. 4)

Of equal or more importance was the new way in which Black women saw themselves. No longer isolated in the United States, they saw themselves as part of a global movement of Black and Brown people united in struggle against the colonial, imperialist, and capitalist domination of the West.

In recent years, the term "Women of Color" has been questioned by many ethnic and racial minority women because the word "color" is not the primary issue for many women who share ethnicity and race. I acknowledge these concerns. The primary focus of this book is intended to transcend terminology and embrace shades of Brown and Black skin color, uniting those of us with shared experiences in the United States.

BLACK FEMINIST THOUGHT

Analyses of psychological, social, and economic conditions are often generalized because they do not consider the ways in which race, class, gender, sexuality, and other facets of identity intersect and produce power dynamics (Collins, 2000; Dill, McLaughlin, & Nieves, 2007). Black feminism scrutinizes these intersecting conditions and creates spaces from which historically conquered knowledges are unveiled, legitimated, and liberated (Collins, 2000; Guy-Sheftall, 1995; hooks, 2000). As such, Black feminist thought provides more complex understandings of interlocking systems of oppression, producing new imaginaries for exposing matrices of power while creating spaces for resistance and possibilities for change.

Black feminist thought and activism has withstood the test of time and continues to be an impressive scholarly and practice paradigm. Women of Color's multilayered activism gives meaning to feminist theory. The first wave of Women of Color's engagement in feminist thought and activism emerged out of the abolitionist movement and culminated with the Suffragists' successful passage of the Nineteenth Amendment. Shirley Yee (1992) detailed how, between 1830 and the 1860s, Black and Native female abolitionists developed a collective feminist consciousness that reflected their particular experiences as Women of Color, as well as the aspects of sexism they shared with White women (p. 151). In particular, free and enslaved African American women created numerous strategies and tactics to resist slavery as a legal institution and racially gendered sexual abuse.

Whether it be Sojourner Truth's much-quoted speech "Ain't I a Woman?" ("Sojourner's Speech," 1851), Anna Julia Cooper's (1892) *A Voice From the South: By a Black Woman of the South*, or Beverly Guy-Sheftall's (1995) prolific Black feminist scholarship *Words of Fire*, Women of Color have aggressively shaped feminist theory and praxis to include issues unique to them. Holding on to Black feminism is a way of protecting a progressive agenda.

Historically, Women of Color have not perceived feminism as relevant to their specific concerns. However, during the first wave of feminism at the turn of the 20th century, Sojourner Truth and a few other African American native women expressed feminist consciousness for Women of Color. Truth (1853/1972), a former slave and abolitionist of the 19th century, spoke out in 1853 in support of the rights of all women: 'I've been lookin' round and watchin' things and I know a little mite 'bout Woman's Rights, too. I come to ... keep the scales a-movin'."

White women involved in the women's movement saw themselves as an oppressed group, which did not lead to the involvement of oppressed Women of Color. One interpretation of this is that the inherent racism of privileged White women prevented them from forming allegiances with Women of Color. It has been the challenge of the modern feminist movement to integrate issues of race, culture, and class into feminist philosophy and feminist therapy practice. Although the feminist movement appeared to exclude men, Women of Color have viewed Men of Color not only as allies but also as leaders in the eradication of oppression (Espín, 1990). White women in the feminist movement also attempted to liken sexism to racism, which caused some resentment among Women of Color (Espín, 1990).

Stone (1979) identified five factors or concerns that contributed to the absence of feminist consciousness and involvement of Women of Color during the mid-20th century: (1) the belief that a focus on sexism would divide the strength of Communities of Color, (2) blatant racism on the part of White women, (3) Black male liberation, (4) the myth of the Black matriarch, and (5) the influence of the Black church to focus on racism rather than sexism. It is important to note that traces of these factors were evident in early and mid-20th-century feminist philosophy and practice and are still observable in current feminist philosophy and practice.

Many of the factors outlined by Stone (1979) continue to provide an understanding of why Women of Color are still skeptical of feminism. In fact, Women of Color are responsible for the multicultural feminist theories that have evolved. Despite diverse concerns and multiple intellectual perspectives, multicultural theories share an emphasis on race as a force in understanding the complexity of gender. The centrality of race, of institutionalized racism, and of struggles against racial oppression is what links the various feminist perspectives within the framework of multiculturalism. In response to challenges from Women of Color, these multicultural theories have begun to be incorporated into the current feminist model (Comas-Díaz, 2015). Although the multicultural approaches are recent additions, Black feminists follow a long-standing approach.

The Black Feminist Movement grew out of, and in response to, the Black Liberation Movement and the Women's Movement. The Black Feminist Movement was formed in an effort to meet the needs of Black women who felt they were being racially oppressed in the Women's Movement and sexually oppressed in the Black Liberation Movement (Guy-Sheftall, 1995). All too often, "Black" was equated with Black men and "women" was equated with White women. As a result, Black women were an invisible group whose existence and needs were ignored. The purpose of the movement was to develop theory that could adequately address the way in which race, gender, and class were interconnected in their lives and to take action to stop racist, sexist, and classist discrimination. This separation from the Women's Movement and Black Liberation Movement was an impetus for consciousness raising toward liberation and eventual healing.

The advancement of Black feminism in the United States developed not only out of Black women's antagonistic and dialectical engagement with White women but also out of their need to ameliorate conditions for empowerment on their own terms. Contributions from Black feminist thinkers and activists such as Francis Beale, Cheryl Clarke, Patricia Hill Collins, bell hooks, Audre Lorde, and Barbara Smith have been foundational in the development of contemporary Black feminist thought. Guy-Sheftall's (1986, 1995) work on Black feminist thought informs a Black feminist approach to therapy and mental health services. The argument that Black women confront both a "woman question and a race problem" (Cooper, 1892, p. 134) captured the essence of Black feminist thought in the 19th century and has reverberated for generations among intellectuals, journalists, activists, writers, educators, artists, and community leaders, both male and female (Guy-Sheftall, 1995). Although feminist perspectives have been persistent and important components of the African American literary and intellectual traditions, scholars have focused primarily on their racial overtones. This tendency to ignore long years of political struggle aimed at eradicating the multiple oppressions experienced by Women of Color resulted in erroneous notions about the relevance of feminism to the Black community during the second wave of the women's movement. Rewriting the history of Women of Color using gender as one category of analysis should render obsolete the notion that feminist thinking is alien to Women of Color or that they have been misguided imitators of White women. An analysis of the feminist activism of Women of Color also suggests the necessity of reconceptualizing women's issues to include sexuality, poverty, racism, imperialism, physical and sexual violence, economic exploitation, decent housing, and a host of other concerns foregrounded by generations of Women of Color.

According to Guy-Sheftall (1995), although Black feminism is not a monolithic or static ideology, and although there is diversity among African American feminists, there are certain constant premises:

- Women of Color experience a particular kind of oppression and suffering in the United States, one that is racist, sexist, homophobic, and classist because of their multiple identities and their limited access to economic resources.
- This multiple jeopardy has meant that the problems, concerns, and needs of Women of Color differ in many ways from those of both White women and Men of Color.
- Women of Color must struggle for racial liberation and gender equality simultaneously.
- There is no inherent contradiction in the struggle to eradicate sexism and racism, as well as the other "isms" that plague the human community, such as classism and heterosexism.
- Women of Color's commitment to the liberation of People of Color and women is profoundly rooted in their lived experience.

In 1977, the Combahee River Collective, a group of mainly Black lesbian feminists, including Audre Lorde, Pat Parker, Margaret Sloan, and Barbara Smith, released a statement that attempted to define Black feminism as they saw it. The collective's work was grounded in a feminist perspective, addressed homophobia, and called for sisterhood among Black women of diverse sexual orientations (Combahee River Collective, 1986). A fundamental belief of theirs was that "Black women are inherently valuable and that our liberation is a necessity not as an adjunct to somebody else but because of our need as human persons for autonomy" (Combahee River Collective, 1986, p. 2). Moreover, they argued that sexual politics is as pervasive in the lives of Black women and other Women of Color as are the politics of class and race, and because race, class, and sex oppression often operate simultaneously in their lives, it is often difficult to separate them. They felt linked to Men of Color in their common struggle against racism and underscored their affinity to them. However, they felt that Black women often struggle with Black men over the issue of sexism.

Patricia Hill Collins's (2000) landmark *Black Feminist Thought: Knowledge, Consciousness, and the Politics of Empowerment* identified the fusion of activism and theory as Black feminism's distinguishing characteristic and analyzed its three core themes: (1) the interlocking of race, class, and gender oppression in Women of Color's personal, domestic, and work lives; (2) the necessity of re-creating positive self-definitions and rejecting denigrating, stereotypical, and externally imposed controlling images (mammy, matriarch, welfare mother, whore), both within and outside of Communities of Color; and (3) the need for active struggle to resist oppression and realize individual and group empowerment (Collins, 2000). The Collins text would further establish, along with Toni Cade Bambara's (1970) *The Black Woman: An Anthology*, bell hooks's (1981) *Ain't I a Woman?*, and Beverly Guy-Sheftall's (1995) *Words of Fire* and (1979) *Sturdy Black Bridges*, a continuous Black feminist intellectual tradition going back to the publication of Anna Julia Cooper's (1892) *A Voice from the South* 100 years earlier. It is both refreshing and enlightening in this most depressing of times to have a historical perspective on an issue that has been with us since slavery.

ORGANIZATION OF THIS BOOK

Postmodern feminisms have warned against creating bipolar categories and remind us of the fluidity of boundaries and the tentative nature of truth. In keeping with this principle, I ask readers to view my structure as a tentative framework that is open to modification and change as new advances in theory, research, and application continue to emerge. To encourage feminist therapists to think comprehensively about the frameworks that inform their work, my goal is to show that coherent connections between specific feminist theories and feminist practices can be drawn. However, individual readers' specific academic and personal experiences influence the organizational framework that is most meaningful to them. I encourage readers to maintain a flexible and open frame of mind as they think about the most useful intersections between feminist theory and feminist therapy that can inform their work.

This book is organized around themes, beginning with an illustration of the mental health experiences of Women of Color, followed by a discussion of recurrent topics and issues that emerge in therapy. Because there is so little evidence of the thoughts and ideas of Women of Color who have been affected by mental illness and of Black feminists—both therapists and thinkers—I use the words of these two groups, taken from interviews, wherever possible to illustrate their experiences and insights.

I have used a "best-fit" approach and embedded the discussion of specific therapeutic approaches at points at which the linkages seemed most logical. Another author with a different set of assumptions and life and clinical experiences may organize these connections in a different manner. For example, some of the Black feminist therapy components that I discuss in the chapters on Black feminist therapy may be relevant to a variety of other chapters and integrative approaches to theory and therapy. Each chapter underscores the necessity of using Black feminist principles in clinical practice with Women of Color.

Chapter 1, "Women of Color's Mental Health Matters: *Mujeres de Color, en la Lucha* (Women of Color, in the Struggle)," locates current psychosocial and behavioral health patterns of Women of Color in the wider historical context of their history of oppression in the United States and their common struggles along with the current social and political atmosphere of oppression. Using the lens of Black feminist analysis, I then provide an overview of the health and mental health conditions of Women of Color and review current economic and social conditions, as well as outcomes.

Chapter 2, "Developing a Black Feminist Analysis for Mental Health Practice: From Theory to Praxis," provides a brief overview of Black feminist philosophies and how they can be translated into healing, wellness, and power in therapeutic services for Women of Color. This chapter also presents the foundational strategies for developing and utilizing Black feminist perspectives in social work practice.

In Chapter 3, "Culturally Responsive Services," I first summarize the empirical literature on Women of Color's mental health service needs, access and utilization issues, and treatment outcomes. Second, I define the concept of culturally responsive services in mental health treatment. Third, I review feminist therapy paradigms and practice principles and their contributions to women's psychology. Moreover, I summarize the evolution of Black feminist therapy, which developed from feminist therapy, and in response to it, in an effort to meet the unique mental health needs of Women of Color. Last, I contend that Black feminist perspectives provide an ideal framework for therapy and counseling services that are aligned with the values, experiences, and worldviews of Women of Color.

Chapter 4, "Understanding Power and Powerlessness in Therapy with Women of Color," acknowledges power as a key concept in Black feminist therapy with many Women of Color. In this chapter, I seek to assist therapists in understanding the many oppressive challenges faced by Women of Color that may add a layer of complexity to their ability to function competently and that often have negative psychosocial consequences (for example, depression, anxiety, strained resources, poverty, poor health outcomes, exposure to violence, and drug addiction). Knowledge of empowerment strategies to enhance psychosocial competence provides a foundation for students or professionals to begin thinking about interventions for this population. For example, empowerment-based perspectives draw on psychosocial competence rather than pathological or maladaptive behaviors (L. V. Jones & Warner, 2011). Thus, interventions in the mental health field should aim to help Women of Color sort out the personal from the contextual by assisting them to recognize how the internalization of socially constructed identities has contributed to their depressive symptoms (C. B. Williams, 2005).

Chapter 5, "Applying Black Feminist Therapy Approaches to Women of Color in Therapy," draws from the practice literature on therapeutic approaches for Women of Color, focus group data I have collected, and my 25-plus years of mental health practice experience. In this chapter, I explore recurrent themes in therapeutic practice with Women of Color, including issues of racism and sexism, guilt and shame, sexual identity and sexual orientation, and economic pressures. Case studies and qualitative data are used to demonstrate how practitioners can fully integrate Black feminist strategies in the engagement, assessment, intervention, and termination stages of the treatment process.

Chapter 6, "Case Illustrations," provides therapeutic practice examples based on my clinical experience, using individual, group, and family modalities that highlight the basic components of Black feminist therapy outlined in Chapter 2. These case illustrations can be used to facilitate clinical supervision, class discussion, role-plays, or other small-group exercises.

Chapter 7, "Claiming Your Connections: An Evidence-Based Psychosocial Competence Group Intervention Grounded in Black Feminism," describes the Claiming Your Connections (CYC) evidence-based group intervention model. The CYC intervention is designed to expand opportunities for Women of Color in mental health therapy to engage in culturally congruent, therapeutic interventions. It hones in on the outcomes of decreasing external locus of control and increasing active coping from a culturally relevant perspective on the basis of the needs and experiences of Women of Color.

Chapter 8, "Black Feminist Therapy: A 21st-Century Imperative," summarizes the findings and insights presented in the book. It provides a concluding discussion to assist practitioners in identifying the benefits and constraints of incorporating Black feminist perspectives into mental health treatment. Moreover, this chapter encourages therapists to re-envision wellness versus illness for Women of Color and engage in radical and transformative mental health practices at the micro, macro, and policy levels of practice.

Non-White women will be the majority of all women in the United States by 2060 (U.S. Census Bureau, 2015). We all have multiple identities that affect our life experiences, how we perceive the world around us, and how we are perceived by others. Our gender, race, ethnicity, class, and sexuality intersect to shape the opportunities and challenges we face at school, work, and home and in the community. Acknowledging and addressing this reality is key for therapists seeking to engage in Black women's wellness work. It requires us as practitioners to systematically analyze Black women's oppressions and liberation processes from a Black feminist perspective.

I conclude with a discussion of key terminology to support readers as they navigate the book.

CHAPTER 1

Women of Color's Mental Health Matters: *Mujeres de Color, en la Lucha* (Women of Color, in the Struggle)

It is a struggle being a Woman of Color in the United States, where race and gender are powerful determinants of life experiences. Many Women of Color today carry the weight of centuries of adversity, beginning with the stark exploitation of African peoples in more than 250 years of slavery and extending through the postslavery era of Jim Crow and into present-day institutionalized racism, sexism, classism, and heterosexism. Throughout these eras, Women of Color's social, political, and economic contributions to the United States have been undercompensated and undervalued.

Compared with White and Asian women, Women of Color are among the most likely to be affected by adverse social, political, and economic conditions such as poverty, underemployment, joblessness, incarceration, homelessness, and lack of access to basic health care. In 2017, Women of Color experienced higher poverty rates and were paid less than their White counterparts for the same work (Institute for Women's Policy Research [IWPR], 2017; U.S. Census Bureau, 2015). When working full time, Black women earn just 62.5 percent of White male median earnings and 87.5 percent of Black male median earnings (IWPR, 2017). The difference is less among women; Black women's median weekly earnings ($671) were 82.8 percent of those of White women ($810). Overall, median weekly earnings of Hispanics ($675) and Blacks ($696) were lower than those of Whites ($911) and Asians ($1,066) (Bureau of Labor Statistics, 2016).

Proportionally, Women of Color are enrolled in college at a higher rate than any other racial–gender group (9.7 percent versus 8.7 percent for Asian women and 7.1 percent for White women). Unfortunately, although Women of Color may be earning degrees at a disproportionate rate, recent data have shown that at all educational levels, Women of Color are concentrated in lower-paying jobs than Black men and White men and women (IWPR, 2017). Moreover, the socioeconomic and employment conditions of Women of Color influence access to health and mental health insurance and, therefore, health care. Women of Color have lower rates of health insurance coverage (approximately 83.5 percent compared with their White female counterparts at 89.8 percent; IWPR, 2017), and when they do receive health care, their quality of care is lower than that of White women and men (Office of Research on Women's Health [ORWH], 2014).

In addition to socioeconomic status, *acculturation*—the process of psychological and behavioral change that people undergo as a consequence of long-term contact with another ethnicity or culture—plays a significant role in the incidence of mental health conditions and access to health care. Discrimination, prejudice, and exclusion (based on language, skin color, economic class, or other factors), perhaps for the first time, present Women of Color (and all People of Color) with the predicament of identifying with a newly acquired "minority" status. This perception can often affect health- and mental health–seeking behavior as well as disparities in receiving efficient and effective care. These economic, educational, contextual, and social inequalities have often exacerbated or even created mental illnesses or concerns among Women of Color (ORWH, 2014).

MENTAL HEALTH

It is important to define the terms "mental health," "mental illness," and "mental health concerns" as used in this book.

- *Mental health* is defined as a state of well-being in which every individual realizes their own potential, can cope with the normal stresses of life, can work productively and fruitfully, and is able to make a contribution to their community. The positive dimension of mental health is stressed in the World Health Organization's (WHO's; 2003) definition of health as contained in its constitution: "Health is a state of complete physical, mental and social well-being and not merely the absence of disease or infirmity" (para. 1).
- *Mental illness* refers to a wide range of mental health conditions—disorders that affect one's mood, thinking, and behavior. A few examples of mental health disorders are depression, anxiety, drug abuse or addiction, schizophrenia, and eating disorders.
- *Mental health concerns* may show up as signs and symptoms that impede one's everyday life, such as feeling sad or down; reduced ability

to concentrate; excessive fears or worries; extreme feelings of guilt; extreme mood changes; withdrawal from friends and activities; problems sleeping; inability to cope with daily problems or stress; alcohol or drug abuse; major changes in eating habits; and excessive anger, hostility, or violence (American Psychiatric Association, 2013). In fact, signs or symptoms of a mental health concern sometimes appear as physical problems, such as an upset stomach, back pain, headache, or other unexplained aches and pains. A mental health concern becomes a mental illness when ongoing signs and symptoms cause frequent stress and affect one's ability to function (WHO, 2003).

WOMEN OF COLOR'S PSYCHOHISTORY

As James Baldwin (2010, p. 154) said, "History is not the past. It is the present. We carry our history with us." Women of Color who possess a spiritual or mystical consciousness know that the past reverberates in the present and the future. Hence, when we speak of mental illness and wellness among Women of Color, we must begin by understanding how the traumatic experiences of slavery have been passed down through the generations. The historical wounds of enslavement, conquest, and colonization continue to have an impact on the psychological health of Women of Color, even if their familial origins are outside the United States. A major link between Latin and Black communities is that both groups were forced to migrate to the United States for economic, political, environmental, and social reasons for the purpose of cheap labor (Gutierrez, 1990). Because they were forced to live in the United States and leave behind their extended families, communities, and culture, they suffered psychic injury, compounded by the patriarchal, racist structure of the United States.

Jenkins (1993) discussed how, under the U.S. slavery system, African American women's "survival was dependent on this oppressive institution, which exploited her biological reproductive capacity, required her to work, care for, and live through others despite her own needs and constant subjection to social male toxic violence, resulting in trauma" (pp. 119–120). During slavery, this role was adaptive for survival, but it also required a connection to the oppressor and a disconnection from the self. For instance, enslaved women were forced to comply with sexual advances from their masters on a regular basis. Consequences of resistance often came in the form of physical beatings, being sold off, and, at times, death. Thus, slave women often dissociated from their sexual and physical selves to survive the demonic conditions of sexual exploitation or violence.

A present-day resonance of this adaptation may be seen in the mythology of the "Strong Black Woman" (SBW) who is selfless and all-giving of her body, her emotions, her skills, and her labor (Mullings, 2006; Woods-Giscombé, 2010). Today, many Women of Color continue to rely on this adaptation for a sense of survival in continuous and unpredictable hostile environments. An example is the online harassment of and threats toward Women of Color. Although not a new phenomenon, the degree to which these are directed at Women and Girls of Color has increased. For instance, racism and sexism can blend together in the mind of the harasser and be displayed as an inseparable whole. The types of statements used and actions taken incorporate the unique characteristics of Women of Color, subjecting each race and ethnicity to its own cruel stereotype of sexuality. As discussed earlier, harassment of African American women may incorporate images of slavery, degradation, sexual availability, and natural lasciviousness, whereas although harassment of Latina women may also include images or microaggressions pertaining to servitude, they may also be seen as hypersexual or hot headed or be sexually fetishized. This subjectivity often creates a continuous state of emotional trauma that disrupts the ability to develop effective coping strategies (Lewis & Grzanka, 2016).

Forms of online harassment can vary, from racialized or sexualized name calling to persistent stalking and outright threats of sexual and personal violence. It remains the case that the wide-open environment that enables creativity and innovation online also enables derogatory and sometimes anonymous speech against which Women and Girls of Color often have no recourse. An Indigenous colleague shared one of her experiences with online harassment via a post on her Facebook page:

> Just read an article of yours re aborigines don't get a free ride. So why when I join a gym or go to any government department they ask if I'm indigenous and to tick a box. As a white person I find this so racist and discriminating. What has joining a gym got to do with my race unless there are some freebies.

She spoke about this posting with rage and frustration, stating, "as an educated and privileged woman you'd think I could 'brush my shoulders off.'" Further referencing the words of the rapper Jay-Z—"If you feelin' like a _____, go and brush your shoulders off/Ladies _____ too, gon' brush your shoulders off/Get, that, dirt off your shoulder"—she responded, "I can't brush it off; it festers." This is one example of the daily harassment Women of Color may experience on social media in regard to their race, gender, or both.

A Woman of Color is socialized to believe that everyone else's well-being matters more than her own. She suppresses her dreams to assist in fulfilling those of others around her; she thrives on being the most obedient, solid rock of a servant possible (Abrams, Maxwell, Pope, & Belgrave, 2014; Beauboeuf-Lafontant, 2009). For instance, many Latina women are also often characterized as submissive, self-denying, and self-sacrificing for the sake of those they serve. In the family environment, the ideal Latina woman is one who places the needs of her children and husband first and asks little for herself in return (Gutierrez, 1990). Experiencing this continuous state of emotional trauma eventually disrupts Women of Color's ability to develop effective strategies to respond to stressful or traumatic events (Abrams et al., 2014).

This cultural bond translates into gender relations and roles, called "machismo" and "marianismo," which call for distinct gender roles for men and women. "Machismo" (similar to male chauvinism) refers to characteristics of the male that include dominance, virility, and independence; "marianismo" refers to characteristics of the female as submissive, chaste, and dependent. Traditionally, the Latino man is the economic provider and the Latina woman is responsible for the domestic roles, most notably, caretaking of the children. Machismo-based family relations can inhibit Latina women from being considered truly equal to Latino men (T. Brown & Smith, 2009). As a result, Latina women can become increasingly alienated from their emotions and cover their humiliation and shame with anger, substance abuse, and depression.

SNAPSHOT OF WOMEN OF COLOR'S MENTAL HEALTH

In recent years, some progress has been made in acquiring a public platform for Women of Color with mental illness. For example, Women of Color celebrities such as Kerry Washington, Taraji P. Henson, Eva Mendes, Alicia Keys, and Gina Rodriguez have shared their personal experiences with mental health issues and stressed the importance of seeking treatment. But there is still a long way to go. The push for health care access under the Obama administration spawned a greater awareness of the role of ethnicity and race in the provision of appropriate mental health services for Women of Color. Until recently, research on mental health services did not consider race or ethnicity (U.S. Department of Health and Human Services [HHS], 2001). The development of research-based recommendations to improve access and utilization has been hampered by the lack of racial and ethnic minority representation in treatment and intervention studies (H. W. Neighbors et al., 2007; Substance Abuse and Mental Health Services Administration [SAMHSA], 2012). Thus, any bearing that race and culture may have on the manifestation, perception, recognition, and salience of psychosocial symptoms and substance abuse risk factors continues to be overlooked in service utilization research (T. A. Davis & Ancis, 2012; Ono, 2013).

According to HHS (2001), Women of Color are 20 percent more likely to report serious psychological distress than their White counterparts. Moreover, they report an average of 4.7 days per month of poor mental health in terms of managing stress, depression, and other emotional problems

(Melfi et al., 2000). Fewer than 9 percent of U.S.-born Latinas and Caribbean American women seek care in mental health settings, and fewer than 20 percent seek such care in general health care settings. Immigrant Latinas and Caribbean American women are even less likely to seek mental health treatment. However, African American women are more likely than Latinas to receive treatment for depression (Alegría et al., 2002).

The fact that mental health symptoms or signs of distress often manifest as somatic symptoms among Women of Color also calls for attention. Research has shown that Women of Color have high rates of poor physical health outcomes as a result of psychological stress, much of which goes undetected. Many poor health outcomes experienced by Women of Color may either be created or exacerbated by repressed anger and stress related to a sense of powerlessness (S. A. Thomas & González-Prendes, 2009). For instance, several independent risk factors have been identified, ranging from physiological factors such as diastolic blood pressure and immune disorders (Artinian, Washington, Flack, Hockman, & Jen, 2006) to psychosocial factors such as chronic stress (Grote, Bledsoe, Wellman, & Brown, 2007) and a lack of social support (Lincoln, Chatters, Taylor, & Jackson, 2007). J. Jackson et al. (2007) have suggested that coping with structural barriers and racial bias may be a common underlying cause of stress-related mental illnesses, such as mood and anxiety disorders (Lawson, Rodgers-Rose, & Rajaram, 1999; Nuru-Jeter et al., 2009; D. R. Williams, 2000). According to Geronimus, Keene, Hicken, and Bound (2007), the psychological and physiological responses to stress experienced by many People of Color over their life course may lead to chronic physical and psychological health problems, such as high blood pressure, heart disease, diabetes, and lupus.

Very little attention has been paid to the prevention and treatment of Women of Color's health, specifically mental health, psychosocial stress, and illness (HHS, 2001). A full understanding of these multiplicative risk factors based on negative health and mental health outcomes is elusive. Compounding the issue is the fact that Women of Color are less likely to seek treatment for mental illness than their White counterparts (Alegría et al., 2002; Matthews & Hughes, 2001; Neal-Barnett & Crowther, 2000). When Women of Color with psychosocial difficulties do seek help, it has traditionally been through informal sources such as family, friends, and clergy (Glass, 2012; Nadeem, Lange, & Miranda, 2009).

Although several outcome studies have examined Women of Color's mental health treatment and the barriers to that treatment, few have explored their experiences and perceptions of these barriers. Research has indicated that racial, gender, class, and sexual identity differences are important factors to consider in the design of mental health treatment services Ehrmin, 2005; HHS, 2001; Institute of Medicine, Committee on Understanding and Eliminating Racial and Ethnic Disparities in Health Care, 2003; Wallen, 1992; Weiss, Kung, & Pearson, 2003), yet little attention has been paid to cultural variations, which may have important implications for strengthening service provision for Women of Color.

Several barriers to treatment engagement for Women of Color with mental illness have been identified. These barriers may include shame and stigma, cultural and language differences, fear and distrust of the treatment system (which is based on White middle-class values and perceptions of [biases against] People of Color), lack of information, and lack of medical insurance and transportation (Bowie & Dopwell, 2013; Choi & Gonzalez, 2005; Nadeem et al., 2009; Snowden, 2001). These barriers often prevent Women of Color from receiving proper support or treatment. Latina and Black women are more likely than White women to report stigma concerns as a reason for not seeking mental health services (Alvidrez & Azocar, 1999; Cooper-Patrick et al., 1997). Similarly, Caribbean American immigrants report concerns about being labeled "crazy" (Schreiber, Stern, & Wilson, 1998), which reduces their willingness to seek and engage in mental health services (Edge, Baker, & Rogers, 2004; Keating, Robertson, McCulloch, & Francis, 2002). This negative perception of help seeking must be eliminated if Women of Color as a community are going to help people who live with mental health disorders to heal—emotionally, physically, and spiritually. As shared by a Woman of Color client during a focus group,

> So, it would help more to reach out to those who are struggling with depression, and have a little compassion about it. Don't put labels on them, you know. Everybody's got a label. "Oh, she crazy" [while motioning with her finger], "He acting just like a crack-head. Oh that's an addict." You know what I'm saying? Or "She's on welfare, you know," or "She ain't never going to be nobody." This stigma got to stop. Stop labeling people with mental illness, and people got to stop accepting labels, too.

If People of Color are not able to take care of themselves, their families, and their communities and find ways to cope in a healthy manner, many of these negative messages are internalized without their being aware of it, causing damage to their spirits.

Another barrier to seeking and receiving counseling identified by Women of Color is the mental health profession's assumption that all women are alike, as are all Women of Color. The danger is that therapists and researchers will overgeneralize and overlook the tremendous within-group variability. Therapists must take into account ways in which Women of Color experience racial, sexual, and economic bias and bigotry and how their experiences may be different from White women's and men's experiences. Moreover, therapists should understand that not all Women of Color experience these oppressions similarly, nor do they manifest the psychological consequences of these oppressions similarly.

Moreover, when Women of Color do seek professional mental health services, they are more likely than others to have reached a crisis point and are more likely to be misdiagnosed by the therapist or provider (Carrington, 2006; T. A. Davis & Ancis, 2012; H. W. Neighbors et al., 2007). In addition, they may prematurely withdraw from treatment because their ethnic, cultural, or gender needs go unrecognized or they are mistreated because of their race or gender (Blazer & Hybels, 2000; C. Brown & Palenchar, 2004; T. A. Davis & Ancis, 2012; H. W. Neighbors et al., 2007). One consistently highlighted shortcoming is that treatment interventions lack cultural relevance and are inadequate to meet the specific needs of Women of Color (Comas-Díaz & Greene, 1994; Institute of Medicine, Committee on Understanding and Eliminating Racial and Ethnic Disparities in Health Care, 2003; L. V. Jones & Warner, 2011; Miranda & Cooper, 2004; HHS, 2001). In fact, President George W. Bush's New Freedom Commission on Mental Health (2003) described in detail the gender, racial, and cultural problems associated with access to and utilization of mental health and drug abuse services, concluding that the higher burden of mental health disability among racial minorities may be attributed to treatment barriers (for example, access to a provider, cost, culturally relevant services).

In addition to culturally endorsed coping strategies, an understanding of specific barriers to therapeutic service utilization will aid researchers and clinicians in developing culturally relevant interventions, as well as treatment engagement and retention strategies that will meet the needs of this growing population. An important goal of practitioners must be to attend to individual and societal stressors, especially those influenced and exacerbated by experiences of discrimination, oppression, and mistreatment in an effort to promote positive mental health outcomes (Borum, 2012; Conner et al., 2010; T. A. Davis & Ancis, 2012; Neal-Barnett & Crowther, 2000; SAMHSA, 2012; HHS, 2001). The conflicted relationship that Women of Color have with the institution of therapy is also noteworthy. For many Women of Color, being in therapy means that they have failed in their role as (super)women. Moreover, Women of Color come to therapy viewing themselves as the problem versus having a problem.

These challenges and barriers may suggest that mental health providers seeking to engage Women of Color in therapy, often referred to as "wellness work," must use sources of knowledge beyond the canon of mainstream psychology. This work requires therapists to engage in a systematic analysis of the oppressions and liberation processes of Women of Color from an ecological perspective. Hence, understanding the intersectionality of Women of Color's identities and perceptions is critical in the therapeutic process. In partnership with the client, the therapist can explore the story of the Woman of Color who is sitting in the room, develop trust, and establish the goals of therapy. This process will help to promote self-actualization, empower self-growth, improve relationships, and reduce emotional suffering (L. V. Jones & Warner, 2011). Hence, a Black feminist therapeutic strategy may help Women of Color redevelop or strengthen their historical identity as a means of empowering them to change the conditions that produce their societal understanding of themselves as failed. Moreover, they engage in a healing process that empowers their sense of self-efficacy in achieving life outcomes and goals.

BEYOND THE DATA

Although history and empirical studies have demonstrated that Women of Color are disproportionately more likely to experience life events that increase their chances of having a mental illness, they raise the following questions: (a) Why do so many Women of Color suffer in silence? and (b) How can mental health counselors engage with them, build trust, and help them with their struggles when they have convinced the world that they are strong and do not need help? To answer these questions, we need to understand how Women of Color have traditionally dealt with mental health struggles. By and large, their struggles involve coping with difficulties in isolation, not reaching out to trusted friends and family members, being afraid to ask for help, being too ashamed to seek help, not knowing where to seek help, neglecting their own needs while taking care of others, hiding behind their pain, dismissing the help that professional treatment could provide because of perceived and real bias, and not being able to access therapeutic service because of a lack of insurance or lack of treatment in their region. Women of Color must come to terms with their sense of powerlessness over mental health issues and accept them as temporary so they can receive an optimal level of support. Women of Color must give themselves permission to heal.

CHAPTER QUESTIONS

1. How might social, economic, and contextual factors influence Women of Color's health and mental health status?

2. What are the barriers for Women of Color who seek professional mental health treatment? How do these barriers resonate with you personally?

3. How does current popular culture affect the mental health awareness of Women of Color and contribute to ending stigma?

CHAPTER 2

Developing a Black Feminist Analysis for Mental Health Practice: From Theory to Praxis

> *The concept of the simultaneity of oppression is still the crux of a Black feminist understanding of political reality and, I believe, one of the most significant ideological contributions of Black feminist thought.*
>
> —Black feminist scholar Barbara Smith (1983, pp. 257–258), in *Home Girls: A Black Feminist Anthology*

Mental health praxis has traditionally been defined by scholars as the unity of theory and practice—the relationship among thought and action, reflective practice, and informed action (Quinlan, 2012; Raelin, 2007; Weiner, 1994). Black feminist praxis goes further in that it incorporates lessons learned from past discrimination, marginalization, and activist engagement into present-day practice with Women of Color. A Black feminist therapeutic meaning of praxis acknowledges that seeking knowledge just to know—but not to understand, apply, and advocate—will not change the structures of oppression in the lives of Women of Color. Rather, Black feminist praxis is about applying one's understanding of the client's experience with any or all oppressions while engaging in affirmative healing practices. Hence, we arrive at a juncture discussed by hooks (1984): There cannot be a Black Feminist Movement in education, employment, or health, including mental health, without a praxis informed by Black feminism. In this chapter, I provide a brief synopsis of the development of feminist therapy, discuss the outgrowth of the Black feminist praxis, and present a Black feminist blueprint for working with Women of Color in therapy.

SYNOPSIS OF FEMINIST THERAPY

Feminist therapy is an integrative approach to mental health that focuses on gender and the particular challenges and stressors that women face as a result of bias, stereotyping, oppression, discrimination, and other factors that threaten their mental health (B. P. Jones, 2003). The therapeutic relationship, based on an authentic connection and equality between the therapist and the client, helps empower clients to understand the social and psychological factors that contribute to their issues, discover and claim their unique identity, and build on personal strengths to better their own lives and those of others (Fulani, 2009). Feminist therapy emerged out of the women's movement of the late 1960s, emphasizing the need to address women's struggles with gender roles that often caused psychological distress (Enns, 1997).

Feminist therapy evolutionists were aware of the pressures of patriarchy and institutional dominance in the therapeutic process. For example, women often experienced denigration and dominance in numerous overtly oppressive and microaggressive ways in the therapeutic relationship as well as through expectations about what male therapists believed the female role ought to be and how it should be developed. These assumptions about women's roles and women's place in the home often hindered women in the therapeutic process, which in turn had a negative impact on their ability to heal from their experienced wounds (Enns, 1997).

In addition, feminist psychology developed as a criticism of psychoanalytic theory. Not only were many psychological theories developed by men, but also the research studies used to test these theories historically included only men. Feminist therapists argued that Freud's theories, such as penis envy and hysteria, were gender biased. Traditional Freudian psychoanalysis is predicated on the male oedipal conflict as the basis for normal psychosexual development, whereas female sexuality is presented from the perspective of biological deficit based on the female gender position as castrated male (Kaslow & Magnavita, 2002).

Feminist therapists strongly reacted to and opposed Freudians' gender biases and demanded alternative psychological theories and therapies that not only helped to understand women's emotional imbalances but also developed women-centered psychology beyond "male norms and behavior" (Nugent & Jones, 2009). It was one of the first times that the legitimacy of the male therapist and male-dominated therapy was brought into question. In particular, feminists attempted to build, and to varying degrees succeeded in building, a nonauthoritarian model for doing therapy in which the client–therapist relationship was not defined by the traditional male–female roles and dominant–passive paradigms. In turn, the focus was on developing egalitarian therapist–client relationships, valuing women's experiences, and redefining mental illness from hysteria to women's reactions to the oppression of daily living. From the midst of these movements, feminist therapy emerged.

Feminist therapy has further evolved in terms of theory, therapeutic techniques, and scope of application. Although feminist therapy initially focused exclusively on women and excluded men, both as therapists and clients, contemporary feminist therapy now includes male clients and therapists and seeks nongendered and culturally equitable ways to approach and interpret behavior (Sharf, 2003).

No single person can be identified as the founder of feminist therapy. The growth of feminist therapy has involved a grassroots collaborative process with input from scholars, researchers, and practitioners (L. S. Brown, 1994). Notwithstanding, several authors made developmental contributions to feminist therapy: Anna Freud, Margaret Mahler, and Karen Horney were among the first to break from the dominant psychoanalytic male views of human development. They offered compelling alternative arguments for concepts such as penis envy, female masochism, and feminine inferiority (Sommers-Flanagan & Sommers-Flanagan, 2004). Many books were highly influential: Helene Deutsch's (1945) *The Psychology of Women*, Clara Thompson's (Thompson & Green, 1964) groundbreaking text *Interpersonal Psychoanalysis*, and Jean Baker Miller's (1973, 1976) works reaffirming feminist psychology, *Psychoanalysis and Women* and *Toward a New Psychology of Women*. Many contemporary theorists such as Judith Worell (Worell, Remer, & Worell, 1992), Laura S. Brown (1994), and Carol Zerbe Enns (1997) have published books that address the impact of feminist theory on practice, assessing both the process and the outcomes. Lyn Mikel Brown and Carol Gilligan (1992) also focused on feminist ethics and boundaries, especially as they relate to anti-oppressive therapy and counseling.

NEXT ERA OF FEMINIST THEORY

The challenge for contemporary feminist theorists and therapists was to move beyond the issues of women who were representative of the majority culture and to consider issues involving race, ethnicity, and class. Black feminist mental health therapists and scholars alike challenged these feminist theorists to be more inclusive of race, class, and sexual orientation (Fulani, 2009; L. C. Jackson & Greene, 2000; C. B. Williams, 2005). For instance, Olivia Espín (1993), a pioneer in the theory and practice of feminist therapy with Women and Girls of Color, has done extensive research, teaching, and training on multicultural and lesbian issues in counseling and therapy. Beverly Greene (1994), Nancy Boyd-Franklin (1991), and Lillian Comas-Díaz (2015) explored the intersection of diagnostic and treatment categories of race and culture, specifically regarding Black American and Latina women. Most Women of Color feminism asserts that many of the other feminist perspectives do not take into account other factors of female diversity, such as race, ethnicity, social class, and sexual orientation, although these dimensions also affect women's lives (Fulani, 2009). Black feminism (also referred to as *Black standpoint*) falls into this category and argues that Black women's social realities, stories, and experiences are invisible, having been overshadowed by a focus on White women's experiences.

Advocates of Black feminist therapy and other Women of Color feminist therapies have issued an urgent mandate to address all forms of marginalization and discrimination beyond gender issues alone (Sparks & Parker, 2000). This mandate proposes that therapeutic processes and methods must reflect the psychological and social realities faced by Women of Color within their cultural contexts (L. V. Jones & Warner, 2011; Sparks & Parker, 2000). Black feminist therapies have been identified as one such method.

BLACK FEMINIST THERAPY

Black feminist therapeutic perspectives are offered as an alternative to traditional mental health frameworks that view Women of Color as "others" (for example, worse, less than) and Whiteness, maleness, heterosexuality, and middle-class status as the norm. These norms have resulted in biased psychological frameworks and therapeutic treatment modalities that consistently fail to acknowledge experiences that differ from dominant patriarchal, White, middle-class perspectives (L. C. Jackson & Greene, 2000; L. V. Jones, 2015). Hence, Black feminist therapy evolved as a means to empower all marginalized women, in particular, Women of Color, who often felt silenced or oppressed by mainstream therapies.

Black feminist therapists propose theories and practice interventions that assist Black women in connecting their personal struggles resulting from the structural constraints of racism, sexism, classism, and homophobia. The Black feminist approach thereby moves Black women's life situations from a model of pathology to one of wellness. Therapeutic frameworks developed from a Black feminist perspective help Women of Color recognize how the internalization of stereotypes and negative notions of Black and Brown womanhood contribute to their psychological symptoms and illnesses (for example, depression, anxiety, low self-esteem, and a decreased sense of mastery and power) (L. C. Jackson & Greene, 2000; L. V. Jones & Warner, 2011; King, 1988; McCall, 2005; C. B. Williams, 2005). The use of the Black feminist perspective in mental health therapy helps Women of Color view their reality from a positive, multilayered (that is, sociocultural, political, and economic) perspective and to more clearly understand their struggles, resilience, and strengths. In addition, the Black feminist perspective offers more nuanced conceptualizations of gender and its intersections with race and ethnicity by incorporating a fundamental understanding of Black women's historical, sociocultural, familial, and developmental heterogeneity. The use of Black feminism as a theoretical and conceptual blueprint in therapy with Women of Color recognizes how historical and current transgressions, particularly the racial and sexual injustices endured by Women of Color over multiple generations, affect them and their families today.

Black feminist thought helps practitioners to remain attentive to equity while carrying out scholarship and practice (L. V. Jones & Harris, 2018). Critical self-reflection and community engagement enhance research processes, and research based on the lived experiences of Women of Color and their communities provides the therapist with more significant data on their continuing efforts toward mental well-being. Black feminist approaches to practice emphasize the sociopolitical and historical roots of contemporary disparities, investigate racism, consider how current practice may inadvertently constrain movement toward equity, and highlight the intersectionality of racial and other axes of injustice (Ford & Airhihenbuwa, 2010; Griffith et al., 2007; C. Jones, 2002; Schulz & Mullings, 2006). Taking a Black feminist standpoint asserts the agency of Women of Color as self-determining people with their own resources for healing. Black feminist praxis looks to metaphors, Indigenous practices, spiritualities, experiences of marginalization and discrimination, and understandings of mental health and wellness to inform therapeutic work with Women of Color.

Black Feminist Therapeutic Blueprint

The complex life experiences of Women of Color and the intersection of their race with gender, sexual orientation, ability, and socioeconomic class increasingly demonstrate the need for professional guidance in therapy (L. V. Jones & Warner, 2011). Many Black feminist therapists and scholars have struggled to systematically delineate the therapeutic components of Black feminist therapy (for example, racial–gender power analysis, gender role analysis, consciousness-raising). Here, I provide a blueprint for the use of Black feminist perspectives in therapy. This Black feminist therapeutic blueprint provides a set of culturally congruent recommendations for therapists, regardless of their race or gender, who seek to increase their awareness, knowledge, and skills in mental health practice with Women of Color, most of which can be applied to all Women of Color. Although the blueprint as I have developed it and the supporting literature place substantial emphasis on therapeutic practice, the general guidelines are applicable to mental health practice in its broadest sense (that is, to all Women of Color and female clients of mental health practice), and hence its utility goes beyond the therapist–client dyad.

The Black feminist perspective is a lens through which mental health therapists can better understand, acknowledge, and intervene with Women of Color on the basis of their life experiences. Black feminist perspective in mental health is derived from sociological and psychological theories for viewing Women of Color's functioning, drawing from fields such as psychodynamic, cognitive, and behavioral psychology and narrative, person-in-environment (ecological and family systems), anthropology, interpersonal, and development theories (Collins, 2000). In addition, in the development and delivery of mental health services, this lens incorporates the client's beliefs, values, and assumptions based on how the therapist experiences and interprets the client's psychosocial realities, challenges, and strengths. This lens represents an intellectual and practical effort that draws on a rich cultural legacy, a racial consciousness, and a history that positions the reality of women at the center of the therapeutic intervention (L. C. Jackson & Greene, 2000).

An assumption of the Black feminist lens is that therapists engage in a process of observing and experiencing Women of Color in their natural environments and in their social, cultural, political, and economic reality. This may be done by becoming culturally aware, scheduling a home visit, attending a religious or cultural event, meeting family, and gaining an in-depth narrative of intersecting identities. To work competently with Women of Color, therapists need to have some familiarity with the culture and lifestyles of the client's specific group—in other words, they need to be culturally aware and competent. Moreover, to do ethical and effective therapy with Women of Color, clinicians need to understand the societal challenges Women of Color face in their lives. Many Women of Color wrestle with several common cultural issues as a result of being Women of Color in a racist and sexist society.

I offer the caveat that I am not attempting here to describe the cultural concerns of all Women of Color. Moreover, I believe that it is important that therapists sensitively assess the degree to which these issues are salient for any particular Woman of Color client with whom they are working (addressed in detail in chapter 4). This enables therapists of all races and cultural backgrounds, both male and female, to place themselves in the standpoint or "eyeglass" of the client. This lens is the primary space from which therapists and clients formulate the therapeutic assessment, treatment plan, and goals. Once therapists are committed to this lens, a shift will occur for both the client and the provider, attitudinally and behaviorally. Consequently, the Black feminist lens helps therapists become more cognizant of the life experiences of Women of Color, more self-reflective about the limitations of their own knowledge and experience, and ultimately more acknowledging of diversity and the experiences of women who have experienced systematic oppression.

The Black feminist therapeutic perspective, like most feminist perspectives, consists of a diverse body of disciplines, theoretical orientations, and therapeutic frameworks that are often integrated within other therapy modalities and change processes (Fulani, 2009). It is a practice perspective through which one can engage the client in a process of restoration and lifestyle change. This perspective includes several factors that are key to carrying out Black feminist therapies. I have organized these factors into two groups: structural components and core components.

Structural Components

Black feminist therapists generally agree about some of the structural components of the therapeutic process. Structural components include macro-level forces and institutional barriers about which the therapist must gain awareness and knowledge, including the therapist's practice location, accessibility, and fees and the client's income, insurance coverage, cultural barriers (for example, stigma, internalized oppression, time, family beliefs), religion, and culture (L. V. Jones & Guy-Sheftall, 2015; L. V. Jones & Warner, 2011). The following sections describe these components.

Location and Time Accessibility. Black feminist therapists start with the premise that therapy services for Women of Color should be readily available, affordable, and accessible. They advocate for therapeutic services that enable Black women to receive effective and culturally responsive mental health services in their communities. Unfortunately, for many Black women with mental health needs, obtaining services in their community is extremely difficult because of barriers such as inaccessibility, cost, clinics not located near public transportation, and the dearth of culturally aware mental health providers. This barrier often leads to an inability for Women of Color to access services or, if they do, to their rescheduling or missing appointments, resulting in poor mental health outcomes. In addition, most mental health appointments are scheduled between 9:00 a.m. and 5:00 p.m.—hours when many clients work. Many may not have a flexible work schedule; as a result, their access to services and compliance are threatened (Hernández-Ronquillo, Téllez-Zenteno, Garduño-Espinosa, & González-Acevez, 2003; Hines-Martin, Malone, Kim, & Brown-Piper, 2009). Gonzalez, Williams, Noël, and Lee (2005) have suggested that easy access to therapy, in terms of travel time between residence and therapeutic services, could enhance their compliance. It has also been suggested (Gonzalez et al., 2005) that counseling agencies and private practices offer flexible hours and that community-based agencies and organizations offer auxiliary services, such as child care, meals, and transportation so that Women of Color can access treatment.

Cost of Therapy. The disparity between those who have insurance and the ability to pay for therapy and those who do not is increasing. Many ethnic and racial minorities do not have insurance and cannot afford to pay the high costs of therapy. For instance, therapy fees in New York, Massachusetts, and

Connecticut range from $150 to $300. Fees in Ohio, Iowa, and Kansas range from $100 to $150. Hoyt and Beard (2009) found that two-thirds of primary care physicians in the United States were unable to obtain mental health care for their patients who needed it, largely because their patients lacked insurance coverage or faced prohibitive barriers to using their coverage, including high deductibles and co-payments. Hence, a careful investigation of the Black client's financial situation at the beginning of the therapeutic encounter is a high priority in Black feminist therapy. Such an inquiry enables the therapist to assist the client in understanding her mental health benefits if insurance is limited or nonexistent. If a client cannot meet the required insurance copay, a sliding scale fee could be negotiated.

Cultural Barriers. Individual attitudes toward and responses to mental illness are affected both positively and negatively by one's family and cultural and ethnic community. The cultural environment influences the meaning that individuals assign to mental illness, what the causes may be, and the degree of stigma surrounding mental illness and treatment. In addition, the environment affects whether individuals seek help and, if they do, from whom, as well as how supportive their families are, the pathways they take to obtain mental health services, and how well they respond to different types of treatment.

The cultural community and its attitudes toward mental illness and treatment can also prevent those in need from seeking help for mental illnesses such as addictions, eating disorders, bipolar disorders, and domestic abuse. This is often the case for Women of Color. For example, a common response by clients in my practice is "I feel uncomfortable talking about problems outside of my family—or even within my family." For many Women of Color, talking about feelings or seeking professional help is considered unacceptable for various reasons, including a sense of disloyalty to their family, admitting or showing that they have a personal weakness, fear of misdiagnosis, and concern that they will be treated by a White therapist who has no understanding of their life experiences. In addition, they are reluctant to seek therapy because "the blues" is something that "you just don't discuss!"

Reliance on Religion or Spirituality. The prominence of spirituality and religion among Women of Color also influences whether they seek traditional mental health treatment. Many people who could benefit from mental health counseling have been taught to rely on faith and prayer rather than treatment from strangers, particularly White strangers, of which many Women of Color view the mental health system to consist. In many instances, seeking counseling is considered a lack of faith in God's divine healing powers. Women of Color also often report that they have been taught that one should endure life's difficulties head on and that their faith should carry them through challenging times. As a result, many Women of Color do not seek out needed care, and when they do seek treatment, they do so at the crisis stage, which is not the most effective way to engage in mental health treatment. Women of Color do not need to limit themselves to an either–or scenario. Black women can engage in pastoral (clergy) care, along with prayer for guidance, along with mental health treatment.

Core Components

Although structural components pertain to the impact of Women of Color's political, cultural, economic, and community contexts, core components pertain to Black women's inner lives. Core components include factors that may assist therapists in understanding and acknowledging the impact of Women of Color's multiple oppressions; for instance, how one struggles with internalized oppression and racial identity. These components include, among others, Black women's experiences and the therapist's ability to value those experiences, to recognize the impact of multiple oppressions, and to demonstrate sensitivity in naming and diagnosing problems in the therapeutic process. I expand on these core components here.

Valuing Black Women's Experiences. To be effective in the treatment of Black women, mental health providers must explore and acknowledge their own values, biases, and cultural and religious beliefs and their potential impact on the ability to maintain an empathetic and therapeutic relationship with Black women. Specifically, therapists must be attuned to diversity and its centrality to the ways in which people's values shape the therapeutic process (Feminist Therapy Institute, 2000). According to Comas-Díaz (2014), feminist therapists must understand the culture and values of their clients—in particular, sex role standards and beliefs about sexuality and homosexuality—and adapt their approach accordingly. For example, what are or were the sex role expectations of the client's family of origin? When presented with a lesbian, gay, bisexual, transgender, or queer (LGBTQ) client, therapists must put aside their personal beliefs regarding what they may deem to be moral or immoral and be tuned into the client's needs. In addition, therapists must possess a willingness to validate clients' feelings associated with the racism, sexism, discrimination, and bias they experience in health, mental health, and social service agencies. It is imperative to provide Women of Color with a safe space in which they can tell their stories and redefine or shape their identified problems without feeling invalidated or dismissed.

At a minimum, feminist therapists working with Women of Color must consistently and consciously monitor their personal behavior (for example, words, body language) along with their thoughts, biases, and values to ensure that they do not unintentionally or unconsciously negatively affect clients.

Feminist therapists cannot limit their awareness training to the clarification of personal values; they must expand their own worldviews by becoming informed about the diverse life experiences of Women of Color. This can be achieved by reading relevant literature, attending continuing education events, and working and living in Communities of Color.

Impact of Internalized Oppression and the Strong Black Woman (SBW). Throughout their lifetime, many Women of Color have absorbed negative messages about themselves and their race through their schools, teachers, classmates, magazines, social media, television, film, and the news media (Gordon, 2008). Although they may be cognizant of institutionalized racism, have strong self-esteem, and exemplify resilience, most Women of Color must rely on their mental fortitude to withstand the everyday racism they face and the related social and economic pressures. Trying to be strong and resilient does not prevent the effects of oppression from diminishing their sense of self-efficacy and self-identity (Gaylord-Harden & Cunningham, 2009).

This construct of mental and physical fortitude, including the SBW schema, has been discussed in various literatures (Abrams et al., 2014; Beauboeuf-Lafontant, 2009; Woods-Giscombe, 2010). In the SBW schema, which has deep historical roots, Women of Color are seen as possessing the ability to assume multiple caretaker roles—for their children, husbands, extended families, and community—along with serving their White bosses (Abrams et al., 2014). In this schema, when many Women of Color experience physical or psychological distress, fear, anxiety, anger, and rage, they feel they have no space or permission to express these feelings. They have internalized the SBW belief and feel they must remain strong and tight-lipped at all costs (Beauboeuf-Lafontant, 2009). If such fear, anxiety, or rage is expressed, Women of Color fret that they may be seen as weak or crazy. Hence, therapists who work with them must understand that although the foundation of internalized oppression may be triggered by a barrage of external pressures (for example, work, money, relationships) (T. L. Brown, Linver, & Evans, 2010), the internalized SBW ideology may be more socially and psychologically distressing (Speight, 2007). This, in turn, can keep Women of Color from seeking therapy, and when they do seek it, they feel reluctant to express their full range of feelings.

In the Black feminist approach, therapists strive to be aware of these and other compounding socialization processes of Women of Color and help them to talk about their feelings along with their hopes and goals. Therapists should also strive to recognize the internalized SBW concept and the subtle ways in which beliefs and behaviors related to gender may affect the life experiences and psychological well-being of Women of Color at various points in their lives. Research has revealed, for example, that when Women of Color are aware of the impact of racism, sexism, and homophobia and affirm their positive attributes and accomplishments, they are less vulnerable to the negative effects of stereotypes (C. B. Williams, 2005).

Sensitivity in Assessing and Diagnosing. As previously mentioned, both psychological assessment and diagnosis, as traditionally practiced, reflect the dominant White culture's concepts of mental health and pathology (K. M. Evans, Seem, & Kincade, 2001; L. C. Jackson & Greene, 2000). That is, the White, male, middle-class, heterosexual, able-bodied viewpoint is the normative perspective. Diagnosis, as traditionally applied, exacerbates the power differential between the therapist and the client. By contrast, feminist assessment and diagnosis embodies values of collaboration, fairness, and phenomenology (Gardner & Enns, 2004; K. M. Evans, Kincade, Marbley, & Seem, 2005).

Assessment in the Black feminist approach is accomplished through a shared dialogue in which the client is considered to be the best expert because no one knows their thoughts, feelings, experiences, anxieties, and struggles better than the individual seeking support. This dialogue includes an understanding of the personal, cultural, social, and political aspects of the client's distress. Matos (2015) posited that assessment must be reframed to capture the unique and complex psychosocial needs of Women of Color, including their experience of historical and societal role conflicts and their coping strategies for surviving complex, simultaneous oppressions. Matos further suggested that when working with Women of Color, feminist practitioners should "think diagnostically" and use a Black feminist perspective in therapy that considers the multiplicity of oppressions experienced throughout clients' lifetimes, ranging from their parents, partners, educators, supervisors, and co-workers to the wider society. In essence, every past diagnosis or assessment, if necessary, must be questioned in terms of its basis and embedded biases, values, and assumptions. Also, every assessment should be made with an open mind. Cultural assessments and diagnostic methodologies encourage a more accurate evaluation of Women of Color's strengths, coping abilities, and resources. In addition, they should apply this understanding to assessments and intervention strategies (L. V. Jones, 2015).

Structural and Core Components as Barriers or Supports

Understanding the factors that fall within the structural and core components may then help therapists to provide services that meet Women of Color where they are, from their perspective, rather than via traditional therapeutic modalities that expect clients to meet therapists where they are. Black feminist therapists may interpret these components in multiple ways. Some therapists may place higher value on one component than another, depending on their theoretical and practice frameworks. In addition, it should be noted that these structural and core components do not mean that all U.S. women of

African descent have the same experiences and respond in the same way. The diverse experiences, personalities, perspectives, educational levels, and cultural and economic backgrounds of Women of Color shape various reactions to the core and structural components and serve as a source of support or as a barrier to one's ability to access and use mental health services.

Foundational Strategies for Healing

In providing therapy to Women of Color, it is essential that therapists assist them not only in addressing the presenting problem, but also in developing problem-solving and coping skills necessary to resist negative cultural messages, thereby helping to alleviate their psychosocial symptoms. These skills include assisting Women of Color in (a) engaging in consciousness-raising about societal oppressions against Blacks and women (and other "isms" if they apply, such as ableism, ageism, and heterosexism); (b) conducting a race–gender analysis; (c) exploring power imbalances; (d) learning constructive assertiveness and active coping behaviors; (e) understanding how societal and political forces affect their well-being; and (f) encouraging social and political action against all oppressions. Hence, interventions must aim to assist Women of Color to separate the personal from the contextual (social, economic, and political forces) by helping them recognize how the internalization of socially constructed identities (for example, mammies, who are seen as innately caring for others at their own expense; Jezebels, considered sexually permissive women; Welfare Queens, for welfare recipients; and Angry Black Women, for women expressing negative emotions) contributes to their emotional difficulties (L. V. Jones, 2008; Roberts, Jackson, & Carlton-LaNey, 2000; C. B. Williams, 2005).

Consciousness-Raising in Therapeutic Treatment. Black feminists articulated a consciousness-raising process to analyze the psychological, social, and political implications of sexism and racism. More specifically, consciousness-raising has assisted with understanding their multiplicative and intersecting oppressive experiences with race, class, sexuality, and other social psychological factors (Guy-Sheftall, 1995). This process was the beginning of a cognitive liberation process that enabled Black feminists to make connections among social structures, racism, and classism in their lives. This knowledge was regarded as necessary in building the Black feminist movement.

Race–Gender Analyses. Although feminist therapists use diverse theories to inform their work, a hallmark of feminist therapy is race–gender role analysis. Black feminist therapists are more inclined to conduct a race–gender role analysis given the importance of understanding their intersecting identities and how people learn and absorb familial and societal norms. There is evidence to support the notion that race and gender shape Women of Color's attitudes, motivations, behaviors, and mental health outcomes (T. L. Brown et al., 2010). In addition, a race–gender role analysis can be an important component of assessment and involves exploring the impact of race and other identity statuses (for example, gender, age, sexual orientation) on psychological well-being. It also involves exploring the costs and benefits of behaviors that are used to cope with one's experiences based on race and gender and engaging in decision making about future skills and behaviors that the client hopes to use (for example, meditation for stress reduction, psychotropic medication for a reduction in anxiety, exercise for relaxation and physical health).

A race–gender role analysis can be conducted by helping clients to (a) identify expectations associated with the various social identities they use; (b) clarify the ways in which these messages and associated behaviors are reinforced, punished, or undermined; and (c) consider the costs and benefits of expectations associated with various social identities and gender roles.

Black feminist scholars note that the use of these tools in therapy reflects (and values) an integrated analysis of racism, sexism, classism, and other "isms," offering a lens on the multiplicity and simultaneity of oppressions and emotional struggles that Women of Color experience (Bowleg, Huang, Brooks, Black, & Burkholder, 2003; Collins, 2000; A. J. Thomas, Witherspoon, & Speight, 2008). It is critical to understand and acknowledge that being both Black and female in a society that values neither identity presents unique challenges.

The construct of gendered racism may prove a useful medium to comprehend the negative experiences linked to one's race and gender. Therapists conducting group or individual counseling with Women of Color should listen carefully for complaints about mistreatment based on race and gender and validate clients' experiences. Particularly because Women of Color might minimize the effects of gendered racist incidents (and not readily discuss them), therapists can, through the use of cognitive–emotional debriefing (allowing one to cope by discussing stressors in one's environment), inquire directly about clients' experiences with gendered racism. It is also important to help clients generate a variety of ways to cope with the pain associated with gendered racism.

Exploring Power Imbalances. In many parts of the country, mental health practitioners have infrequent contact with Women of Color and are therefore incognizant of the powerlessness that Women of Color face. Hence, it is necessary for therapists to broaden their thinking about what it means to have power, to feel powerless, and to empower. Moreover, while addressing issues of powerlessness, therapists must simultaneously understand the consequences of these power imbalances for their clients and intervene from perspectives that meet the complex psychosocial needs of Women of Color (L. C. Jackson & Greene, 2000; Shonfeld-Ringel, 2000). Power imbalances may occur when a person with authority or dominance over another engages in advocacy and violent or nonviolent direct action in an effort to build their power before they are willing to enter into a negotiation process, for example, when a supervisor attempts to assert power by talking over a supervisee or a spouse or partner asserts power through physical violence within the relationship.

Black feminist therapy is grounded in an analysis of power dynamics that facilitates an ongoing examination of how larger social, economic, and political forces negatively affect the lives of Women of Color. The personal is political, and the political is profoundly personal, especially for Women of Color, because both reflect the actions and values of the larger society that control necessary resources. Waldegrave, Tamasese, Tuhaka, and Campbell (2003) stated that "therapy can be a vehicle for addressing some of the injustices that occur in society. It could be argued that in not choosing to address these issues, the therapist may be inadvertently replicating, maintaining, and even furthering, existing injustices" (p. 4).

According to Browne and Mills (2001), empowerment allows for "the gaining of power by an individual, family group, or community" (p. 23). When therapists embark on empowerment work with clients, they assume a position of powerlessness on the part of the client. People who occupy powerless roles in more than one area of their life face double victimization, and thus empowerment may require targeted or expanded strategies that are not appropriate for those who are not in such positions (Pinderhughes, 2017). As double victims, Women of Color may have to work twice as hard to develop coping strategies, but it is possible that if one powerless role is linked with another powerless role, then modifications to one role may help to change the other (Gutiérrez, 1990; Pinderhughes, 2017). For example, Women of Color face double victimization as a result of racism and sexism; hence, empowerment is a process of increasing personal, interpersonal, and political power so that Black women become motivated and encouraged to improve their overall well-being.

In developing empowerment-based, culturally congruent interventions targeted to Black women, methods must be structured so that clients can experience themselves as competent in the context of a supportive environment (L. V. Jones, 2015). Empowerment techniques that enable people to experience themselves as competent, valuable, and worthwhile—both as individuals and as members of their family, community, workplace, and cultural group—help to create a sense of control in their lives. Effective empowerment strategies require therapists to become vulnerable by using strategies that eschew power derived from their position as expert or from membership in a particular cultural group, as well as by avoiding stereotypes (Pinderhughes, 2017).

Providing effective therapy services aimed at increasing positive mental health outcomes for Women of Color experiencing double and triple oppressions should be a major goal for therapists. These services differ from traditional medical models of stress and other related mental health disorders among Black women. Knowledge of empowerment strategies to enhance competence provides a foundation for mental health professionals to begin to think about interventions for this population.

CASE ILLUSTRATION OF THE ENGAGEMENT PROCESS: RACE–GENDER AND RACE–POWER ROLE ANALYSIS TECHNIQUE

As previously mentioned, a race–gender and race–power role analysis allows Women of Color to recognize how expectations—their own and others'—affect their thoughts, actions, and feelings. Women of Color are encouraged and supported to keep those gendered behaviors they truly value and learn to discard those they do not.

Here, I present the case of Trisha, who has sought out therapy and counseling for her depressive symptoms of irritability, loss of appetite, feelings of hopelessness, and constant crying at night. She was referred to Naomi, who is part of a Black feminist therapeutic consortium. Naomi conducts an initial assessment with Trisha. As with all of her clients, Naomi bases her assessment on the philosophical stance on which Black feminist praxis is based—that race, gender, sexuality, and cultural role socialization inform psychosocial health. Therefore, the intake interview is very thorough. It includes the following information: gender, age, race, sexuality, ethnicity, nationality, culture, the family of origin's similarities to and differences from the cultural group, immigration status, occupation, class, religion or spirituality, languages spoken, roles of family members (including significant extended family), educational background, history of child abuse (physical or sexual), history of adult physical or sexual abuse (including rape and date rape), and substance abuse. After the intake assessment, Trisha reveals, "I feel weak and I can't do anything right. I hear this from my boyfriend, my mother, and my colleagues. I'm a failure." Naomi begins the conversation by initiating a race–gender role analysis with Trisha.

Naomi begins by explaining to Trisha her own beliefs about race, gender, and power roles and how they affect Women of Color. These beliefs include the basic Black feminist therapy tenets—that the personal is political, the therapeutic relationship is egalitarian, women's experiences are valued, and therapy empowers clients. Naomi begins the analysis by telling Trisha that she wants to get a better idea of how she has been affected by societal demands by means of a race–gender and race–power role analysis. This allows Trisha to start to separate her goals and expectations for herself from societal goals and expectations. In addition, Naomi will learn more in-depth, specific information about Trisha's worldview (how she sees and operates in the world as a Woman of Color). This will be helpful in preventing Naomi from making assumptions and overidentifying with Trisha. Trisha engages in the process of sharing her own story with Naomi.

Before the end of the intake assessment, Naomi assists Trisha in developing a wellness toolbox. These are activities that Trisha can use fairly easily to reflect and get a quick mood boost.

Naomi informs Trisha that she can include any strategies, activities, or skills readily available to her. Naomi states,

> The key to overcoming depression is to start with a few small goals and slowly build from there. Draw upon whatever resources you have. You may not have much energy, but you probably have enough to take a short walk around the block or pick up the phone to call a loved one.

Trisha nods in agreement and thanks her for listening to her story of anger, sadness, and disappointment.

WELLNESS TOOLBOX

A wellness toolbox may include strategies, activities, or skills that provide one with a quick mood boost or simply help one relax. The more tools that are available for coping with stress or symptom alleviation, the better. Clients should try to implement a few of these ideas each day, even if they are feeling well:

- Keep stress in check. Not only does stress prolong and worsen depression, but it can also trigger it. Clients should figure out all the things in their life that stress them out. Once they have identified their stressors, they can make a plan to avoid or minimize them.
- Eat a healthy diet, and exercise daily. A balanced diet that includes fruits and vegetables can boost clients' mood and make a difference in their energy levels. Clients can take a long walk, ride a bike, or work in their garden—every minute counts!
- Visit friends or family. Often, when people are feeling low or anxious, they feel more comfortable sinking into their shell, but being around people they enjoy and love may make them feel better.
- Make a phone call to a family member or good friend. Clients can share what they are going through with the people they love and trust and ask for the help and support they need. These people do not have to be able to fix the problem; they just need to listen.
- Avoid alcohol and drugs. If clients are using alcohol and drugs to cope, they could be making their symptoms worse, both while they are using them and in the long run. Clients should be careful with mixing alcohol or drugs and medications; it can be deadly.

- Sleep well. Mental health problems typically involve sleep problems. Whether clients are sleeping too little or too much, their mood will suffer. Clients should get on a better sleep schedule, aiming for at least eight hours a night.
- Practice relaxation techniques. Clients may be surprised by how much simply relaxing reduces stress. A daily relaxation practice can help relieve symptoms of depression and boost feelings of pleasure. Clients can try taking a hot bath and practicing yoga, meditation, or deep breathing exercises.

SAMPLE RACE–GENDER–POWER ROLE PROCESS

Below, I outline sample race-gender-power processes that can be used with Women of Color in therapy. These processes may help Women of Color uncover how race, gender, and power relations affect their identified problem or issue as well as assist in the identification of solutions.

1. Have the client identify the race–gender and race–power role messages she has received. Frame them in the context of being a Woman of Color. In addition, have the client review current definitions of power and choose one that she believes best describes her own definition.
   a. Have the client identify how socialization, societal expectations, and external and internalized forces such as sexism, racism, ageism, and heterosexism have shaped who she is today.
2. Have the client identify the effects and mental health symptoms that impede her daily functioning as a result of the race–gender and race–power role messages she has listed in step 1. Both positive and negative consequences should be explored.
3. Have the client identify the external race–gender and race–power role messages she has internalized.
4. Review with the client the strategies she has historically used to exert power and possible alternative strategies. Discuss ways in which these strategies empower her.
5. Have the client decide which internalized self-imposed and external messages she would like to keep and which she wants to discard. Because the client has identified the benefits and drawbacks of these messages, she will be ready to let down her guard and dive deeper into the underlying therapeutic concerns.
   a. Have the client do a cost–benefit analysis of the different self-empowerment strategies and then decide which strategies she wants in her own toolbox.

TOWARD A BLACK FEMINIST BLUEPRINT

Feminist theory creates a therapy that serves as a way station; it can be one place, although not the only place, in which a person learns to value connection, loses the shame of psychosocial wounds, and becomes accustomed to being the focus of good-quality attention. Therapy fails as an instrument of feminist transformation when it does not to attend to the ways in which everyday connections among and between members of oppressed groups are undermined by patriarchal oppression. As discussed earlier, Black feminist therapy is one such method to support the field of mental health in serving underserved populations such as Women of Color.

Black feminist therapy can be viewed as a beacon in mental health practice, not only in helping to establish therapeutic relationships but also in motivating a political movement to combat the complex and multiple oppressions and stressors faced by Women of Color. Black feminist practice methods can assist Women of Color in consciousness-raising to reconstruct their perception of themselves. It can also help them gain a sense of understanding of their problems (for example, to learn not to blame themselves for their problems, as society often does), reject socially induced shame and degradation, and develop strategies to achieve their goals and live with a sense of dignity and power. Moreover, this perspective can assist therapists in cultivating modes of empowerment that Women of Color can use to develop positive mental health outcomes. These can include helping Women of Color realize their potential in their work and family lives, in personal relationships, and in the political arena of self-advocacy and deinstitutionalization. Therapists can help Women of Color develop positive coping strategies, a better quality of life, and a healthy lifestyle (Thomas & González-Prendes, 2009). Ultimately, the Black feminist therapeutic blueprint, as described in this chapter, can promote equity and social justice for Women of Color and provide an invaluable framework for therapeutic practice with and research with all oppressed groups.

CHAPTER QUESTIONS

1. Discuss the evolution of feminist therapy and the offshoot of Black feminism.

2. What principles distinguish Black feminist therapy from feminist therapy?

3. What are some similarities and differences between feminist and Black feminist theory and therapy?

4. Reflect on and discuss Black feminists as a lens in therapy:
   a. Is there a core component of Black feminist therapy that resonates with you personally or professionally?
5. How do power, powerlessness, and empowerment play a central role in therapy with Black women?

CHAPTER 3

Culturally Responsive Services

I am not free until all women are free, even if we do not share the same experiences.

—Audre Lorde (1981, p. 10)

One of the central problems confronting those of us who attempt to teach, write, and practice psychotherapy from non-White, non-middle-class, and otherwise "alternative" ideologies is how to center our work in the lives of those we serve. In large measure, many of us have learned a particular perspective on the therapeutic process and have been taught to assess, analyze, and apply treatment using generalizable approaches. Thus, we face two important and difficult questions:

1. How do we situate the experiences of those who do not fit within the norm or do not reflect the normative White culture at the center of our practice frameworks?
2. How do we center our discussions of culture to keep the focus on the Women of Color and other People of Color we serve so that they are not further oppressed?

I have come to understand that this is not merely an intellectual process of questioning, nor is it merely a question of adaptation to existing therapeutic models. Rather, it is a question of how to reenvision, develop, and implement therapeutic interventions from a perspective that considers the unique differences of the client without imposing the values, notions, and perspectives of the White European American middle-class norm of the mainstream mental health community of scholars and practitioners.

What I strive to do in my own practice is to address the intersections of race, gender, sexuality, disability, and class through an approach that is culturally aware of and responsive to the needs of traditionally underserved populations, in particular Women of Color. In 20 years of conducting research and working with Women and Girls of Color who experience psychosocial stress and related stressors and mental health disorders, I have listened to, and heard from, many women eager to share their stories of distress, violence, anxiety, addiction, and the blues. I must say that this is not an easy task. However, the experience has provided me with a firsthand understanding of their challenges and strengths and has assisted me in heeding feedback regarding what type of therapy (for example, psychoanalytic, cognitive, interpersonal, feminist, Afrocentric) is most helpful for each individual. I have learned to be *culturally responsive*, which I define as being able to identify bias in oneself and being sensitive to systems that contribute to the positive and negative reinforcement of that bias. For instance, if a mental health therapist comes from a privileged background, they are sensitive to, and have a raised consciousness about, the cultural, ethnic, and racial differences related to that educational and socioeconomic position. Being culturally responsive means confronting personal fears, challenging ignorance, and exploring issues that cause mental health practitioners to engage in power warfare with their clients.

Moreover, the practice of being culturally responsive in mental health therapy involves being competent regarding one's own intersecting identities (race, gender, religion, class, sexuality, and so forth) and recognizing the effects that external structures and institutions have on the ability of Women of Color to function from a positive mental health standpoint. It is also the process of acknowledging that there is no one-size-fits-all solution and that mental health practitioners should draw on the psychosocial realities and possibilities of every individual client who engages in therapy. Finally, it means continuing to grow through each experience and interaction. In this chapter, I summarize the research literature on Women of Color's mental health services utilization issues and treatment outcomes, provide an overview of the literature on culturally sensitive mental health care, and discuss methods for developing culturally responsive mental health services for Women of Color.

MENTAL HEALTH SERVICES UTILIZATION AND TREATMENT OUTCOMES

The availability of and access to quality services directly affects all aspects of Women of Color's mental health care. For many of those who have poor mental health outcomes as a result of the burdens of psychosocial stressors, accessing treatment services can be critical in preventing chronic onset and improving the quality of their lives. Women of Color's underutilization of professional therapeutic services, and their accompanying increase in psychosocial burden because of their unmet needs, has been well established in the mental health literature (Comas-Díaz, 2012; J. Jackson et al., 2007; McGuire & Miranda, 2008; Institute of Medicine, Committee on Understanding and Eliminating Racial and Ethnic Disparities in Health Care, 2003; HHS, 2001). In 2001, the U.S. Surgeon General released a report titled "Mental Health: Culture, Race, and Ethnicity" that documented significant differences in mental health services utilization between non-White Hispanics and racial–ethnic groups by gender (HHS, 2001). The reasons for underutilization are complex and based on historic and ongoing inequalities (Cummings & Druss, 2011; Lee, Matejkowski, & Han, 2017; McGuire & Miranda, 2008; Whiteford et al., 2013).

When Women of Color seek out professional mental health services, they (a) are less likely than White women to obtain professional care; (b) may delay or withdraw from treatment early because their ethnic-, cultural-, or gender-related needs go unrecognized or are not respected; (c) are more likely than White women to have reached a crisis point; (d) are more likely to be misdiagnosed; (e) are not as likely as White women to receive effective, state-of-the-art treatment; and (f) are more likely to use psychiatric emergency services (Alegría, Atkins, Farmer, Slaton, & Stelk, 2010; Blazer, Hybels, Simonsick, & Hanlon, 2000; L. C. Jackson & Greene, 2000; Snowden, 1999; HHS, 2001).

One consistently highlighted reason for treatment underutilization is that therapeutic treatment models are culturally inappropriate or inadequate to meet Women of Color's specific needs (Comas-Díaz, 2010; Greene, 2000; L. V. Jones & Warner, 2011). Woods-Giscombé and Lobel (2008) asserted that mental health systems and treatment models are based on racist, patriarchal concepts of mental health, and new models must be developed to accommodate the pressing needs of women across all racial backgrounds. They suggest that the prevention and treatment of psychosocial distress among Women of Color requires practitioners to use strategies that are based on culturally responsive, racially and culturally affirming mental health paradigms that emphasize clients' strengths and recognize the deficits in their environments.

Culturally Responsive Services

The field of mental health is faced with the critical task of providing culturally responsive services that meet the complex and unique psychological needs of Black, Hispanic, Asian American, and Native American women, which have traditionally been overlooked. In the past two decades, attention has become focused on the needs of non-White racial, cultural, and ethnic groups through the cross-cultural practice and research literature. One goal of this new stream of research and practice is to rethink therapeutic frameworks and adapt existing practice models to serve all women, including Women of Color (Comas-Díaz, 2010; Lum, 2011; McGoldrick, Giordano, & Pearce, 2005; Pinderhughes, 1989; D. W. Sue & Sue, 2013). In short, cross-cultural practice efforts equip practitioners with cultural knowledge about race, gender, and class and are aimed at increasing cultural literacy to improve the level of understanding that mental health practitioners bring to their work with multicultural clients (Husband, 2000). Although this focus is a step toward cultural sensitivity, it overlooks the importance of developing and using therapeutic interventions that reflect the lived experiences of people who differ from the traditional White, middle-class norm. Hence, culturally responsive mental health interventions incorporate skills and attitudes to ensure that they are effectively addressing the needs of Women of Color and their diverse values, beliefs, and sexual orientations in addition to backgrounds that vary by race, ethnicity, religion, and language.

This notion of sensitivity or competence regarding another is predictably American; in the words of Ruth Dean (2001), being culturally sensitive is "positioned in the metaphor of American know-how" (p. 624). This position is consistent with the belief that knowledge brings control and effectiveness and that these should be achieved above all else. I question the notion that one can become sensitive to, or competent in, the culture of another (Goldberg, 2000). Once we presume to know about another, we have appropriated that person's culture and reinforced our own dominant, egocentric position. I propose that mental health practitioners discard the goal of competence and replace it with a state of mind in which they are interested and open but always tentative about what they understand and cognizant that it is difficult, if not impossible, for anyone to fully know or understand another's culture.

Practitioners must instead maintain an awareness of their lack of competence but at the same time adopt a position of responsiveness (as discussed earlier) to the needs of those who are culturally different from the European American norm. In this framework, the client is the expert, and the practitioner, therapist, or mental health counselor seeks knowledge about the client and tries to understand the client's life experiences and unique sociocultural struggles. This practice approach is based on the notion that culturally responsive treatment is ever evolving and that practitioners and mental health care systems must continue to improve their approach to treatment, leading to improved quality of service delivery. Furthermore, this approach allows mental health therapists to pivot from the center (the White middle-class norm) to the experiences of Women of Color, thereby providing culturally responsive therapeutic services. The goal is for therapists to acknowledge, accept, and value the racial, gender, and cultural differences that Women of Color bring to the treatment process and thereby develop culturally responsive interventions. In other words, therapists obtain the knowledge and skills that enable them to appreciate, value, and celebrate similarities and differences within, between, and among Women of Color.

It is not surprising that many professional organizations are now calling for culturally responsive mental health care models (Fortier & Bishop, 2004;

National Association of Social Workers, 2015; National Center for Cultural Competence, 2009; Pistole, 2004; Whaley & Davis, 2007). Requests for culturally responsive interventions grew out of therapeutic process concerns for racial and ethnic minority group populations (that is, African Americans, American Indians and Alaska Natives, Asian Americans, and Hispanics) with respect to issues such as lack of ethnic practitioners, misdiagnoses, racism, sexism, and client mistrust of providers. At the beginning of the 21st century, these concerns were prompted by the growing diversity of the U.S. population, which necessitated changes in the mental health system to meet the various needs of People of Color. In addition, the importance of culturally responsive services has gained support from federal initiatives focused on addressing racial and ethnic minority health and mental health disparities. These initiatives include strategic plans addressing the dearth of research literature, career development programs for researchers from underrepresented groups, requirements for enrolling minorities in clinical trials, and, most notably, the establishment of the National Institute on Minority Health and Health Disparities, which was created in 2000 to lead scientific research to improve minority health and reduce health disparities.

Culture Defined

To discuss the concept of cultural responsiveness, it is necessary to first define "culture." The 10th edition of *Webster's New World Dictionary* (Neufeldt & Guralnik, 1999) defines *culture* as "ideas, customs, skills, arts, etc., of a people or group, that are transferred, communicated, or passed along by the integrated pattern of human knowledge, belief, and behavior that depends upon human capacity for learning and transmitting knowledge to succeed" (p. 282). Membership in cultural categories can be assigned according to particular aspects of identity, such as race, ethnicity, class, age, gender, or sexual orientation or identity. Cultural categories are often treated as though they are monolithic, with defining characteristics that endure over time and in different contexts. In this definition of culture, cultural responsiveness involves learning about the history and shared characteristics of different groups and using this knowledge to increase understanding in an effort to build interventions with clients. However, in more contemporary views, culture is also described as socially constructed: "It is always contextual, emergent, improvisational, transformational, and political; above all, it is a matter of languaging discourse" (Laird, 1998, pp. 28–29). If one starts with this view of culture, then the prospect of becoming culturally responsive takes on a different meaning. How does one become competent at something that is continually changing?

Providing culturally responsive therapeutic services involves applying knowledge of how culture influences the therapist's health beliefs, health practices, and practice skills throughout the intervention process. Moreover, it involves a complex combination of knowledge of diverse cultural practices and worldviews, reflective self-awareness of one's own cultural worldview, attitudes about cultural differences, and skills in cultural assessment. Although practitioners may achieve a certain degree of competence in cultures other than their own, it is next to impossible to become totally culturally responsive to all cultures (Eubanks et al., 2010).

Implementation of this responsiveness to Women of Color is influenced by practitioners' level of knowledge of the client's cultural health beliefs and practices, by their reflection on their own attitudes, by their skill in culturally responsive assessment (Eubanks et al., 2010; Meleis & Hattar-Pollara, 1995; WHO, 2000), and by their ability to implement culturally responsive interventions. In other words, culturally competent practice with Women of Color demands that service providers and practitioners at minimum educate themselves about the multiple identities and the resulting diverse and unique circumstances that define Women of Color. In addition, service providers must be willing to intervene at multiple systems levels, that is, micro (individuals, groups, and families), mezzo (neighborhoods and communities), and macro (society and institutions), even though contact with the person may have been initiated at the micro level (for example, seeking therapy or counseling services). Described next are three practitioner-level proficiency exercises that can help mental health practitioners develop cultural responsiveness and a culturally responsive practice with Women of Color.

Internal Reflection. This exercise engages practitioners in a process of self-reflection focused on their values, personal beliefs, and patterns of bias and how they may shape their actions when providing culturally responsive therapeutic treatment to Women of Color. In this step, practitioners not only observe and learn about the social, emotional, and cultural contexts of the client, but they also engage in a process of self-reflection. Self-reflection regarding personal, institutional, internalized, and subtle forms of bias is a conscious self-examination and in-depth exploration of one's own stereotypes, prejudices, and assumptions about individuals who are different from oneself, an important step in learning to be culturally responsive. In addressing cultural awareness, practitioners must ask the question, "Am I aware of any biases or prejudices that I may have toward Women of Color, or do I have any subconscious or subliminal biases or prejudices toward People of Color, particularly women?" A practitioner's personal beliefs and biases about People of Color in general or Women of Color in specific can lead to poor treatment, misdiagnosis, and overmedication. For example, Women of Color are at a higher risk of misdiagnosis for psychiatric disorders and may therefore be treated inappropriately with drugs (Institute of Medicine, Committee on Understanding and Eliminating Racial and Ethnic Disparities in Health Care, 2003).

Moreover, internal reflection often leads to an awakening of emotions that may result in resistance to change. Self-reflection forces practitioners to confront their habits, beliefs, routines, and values by questioning everything about their identity. This process is important not just to mental health practitioners but to all providers in the fields of health and social services because it is the process by which people "think with a purpose"—that is, think about an experience and evaluate it with the purpose of improving their understanding and future behavior.

Knowledge Building. Cultural knowledge building about U.S. Women of Color involves seeking a sound knowledge foundation with the goal of not only understanding clients' cultural experiences, beliefs, and attitudes, especially when their views differ from those of the practitioner, but also developing a respect for them. Emphasis is given to a genuine willingness and desire to learn about other cultures rather than doing so simply as a practice requirement. For example, the provider then thinks about his or her global understanding of race or gender and works with the client to put observed behaviors into perspective.

In obtaining cultural knowledge, it is critical for practitioners to understand that there are marked differences within and across Women of Color and all their diversity. Women of Color are quite heterogeneous, with variations in ethnicity, sexual identity, gender, class, educational and cultural backgrounds, personalities, values, religious beliefs, and experiences.

Cultural Assessment. In a cultural assessment, the therapist collects relevant cultural data regarding the client's presenting problem or problems and performs an assessment in a culturally responsive manner (Campinha-Bacote, 2008). The goal of a cultural assessment is to explore the client's explanation of her difficulties. Again, I emphasize that Women of Color are not monolithic; they have different values, beliefs, rituals, and customs than their providers (even different from those who may have the same skin color as them, including as a result of class or access to resources), but just because they are different, they should not be seen as "wrong." Rather, the cultural focus of assessment entails examining the sociocultural, ethical, and sociopolitical features that are uniquely situated on the health and wellness continuum. The common assessment question that leads to this first step is "Tell me your story." In my own practice, I follow this question with open-ended questions such as those that follow to elicit the details of the client's experiences for the assessment process:

- What do you think has caused your difficulties?
- Has the cause of your difficulty become a common difficulty in your life? In your family's life?
- What do you fear most about your difficulties?
- How do you cope? Did you learn these coping skills from your family or elsewhere?
- Who offers you emotional support?
- What kind of treatment do you think you should receive?

- Do you have any preferences for a female or male therapist?
- What are you looking to receive from mental health treatment?
- Would you prefer a bilingual therapist?

After listening carefully to the client's responses, I then decide whether any intervention is necessary. One of the challenges practitioners face is to recognize that just because they know how to intervene does not mean that it is appropriate for them to do so in all cases. The practitioner performing the assessment needs to understand the meaning of the culturally desired behaviors and identify ways to accommodate the client as much as possible under the circumstances.

CASE STUDY OF CULTURALLY RESPONSIVE THERAPY

Camile, a 19-year-old woman of European, Jamaican, and Indian descent, has been referred to her local university's counseling center for academic probation and problems at her dorm. Camile is an international student from Jamaica who has had little contact with the Jamaican community or other family since arriving at college. She complains that her parents do not send her money or buy her things. She was upset last month that her mom did not come to family day at the college. During the end of the previous school year, which was Camile's freshman year, her drinking increased dramatically, usually with binges on the weekends. She also got into squabbles with her dorm mates. The resident director (RD) referred her to the counseling center out of concern for her drunken outbursts and concerns about her isolation.

Mrs. Christopher says, "Afternoon, Ms. Harris, or should I call you Camile?"

Camile responds, "Camile is fine."

The therapist picks up on Camile's accent and says, "I picked up an accent; are you from the Caribbean?"

Camile responds, "Yes, ma'am, I'm an international student from Jamaica."

Mrs. Christopher responds, "What a beautiful island; it must be hard to be so far from home. Do you have family or friends in the U.S.?"

Camile says, "No, Miss. Well, actually, I have family in the Bronx, but I have not seen them since last year."

Aware that Camile is feeling uncomfortable with the process, Mrs. Christopher remembers her conversation in class about engagement with People of Color and shifts her tone and approach to seeking a better understanding of Camile's reason for referral. Mrs. Christopher asks, "Do you know why the dean of students asked you to seek out counseling services?"

"Miss, I don't want to waste your time, nothing's wrong with me, my RD just thinks I'm drinking too much, but nothing's wrong with me." Camile becomes a bit teary-eyed.

Mrs. Christopher says, "I know nothing is wrong with you, but sometimes we don't feel good and it's useful to talk to someone. What do you think?"

Angrily, Camile shrugs her shoulders and replies, "All of my dorm mates say I don't talk like them, listen to their music, or eat their food. I hate it here, and my father just says, 'You're there for an education, not for friends.' The Black guys don't even look my way. One guy said in class that I talk funny. I was so embarrassed."

Mrs. Christopher looks directly at Camile and says, "Well, you sound just fine to me." She asks, "Did your parents go to college in the States?"

Camile says, "Nah ma'am, they've never been to the States, they didn't go to college."

Although Mrs. Christopher is a woman of European descent, she decides to use this opportunity to engage with Camile by using personal disclosure in hopes of finding similar ground. Mrs. Cristopher replies, "Maybe they don't understand the importance of social life on campus, as well as how it can be difficult to adjust to college life. While I'm not Jamaican, my parents were similar, so I understand. I would ask them to attend events or just wanted to talk about roommate difficulties. They just said I need to stop complaining and focus on my studies."

Camile feels comfortable opening up and shares, "Maybe there is something wrong with me. . . . I tear up morning and night, I'm always tired and can't focus. That's not me."

Mrs. Christopher has tuned in to Camile's adjustment issues as an international student and as a Black female student on a predominantly White campus. Camile expresses a sense of relief and even smiles when Mrs. Christopher says, "I don't think anything is wrong with you; this is normal for college student adjustment, you're going to be OK. Maybe I can help you become socially connected in ways that are good for you, so that you don't have to use alcohol to cope any longer." Camile nods in agreement.

Camile further opens up, sharing that she feels as though nobody understands her. She states that she used to be happy that she could "pass" as African American, because most of her relatives were "good for nothing." Mrs. Christopher replies, "Camile, maybe your cultural identity is something we can discuss if you would like to meet weekly for some time. What do you think about that?"

Camile smiles and says, "Sounds good to me." They schedule an appointment to meet the following week. After the session, Mrs. Christopher sits down and writes a list of follow-up items:

- Reach out to Mrs. Windsor in the Caribbean Student Association.
- Discuss general workers' knowledge of Jamaican cultural beliefs and challenges in supervision with respect to mental health and well-being that affect female students.

- Offer support groups to provide a safe place for Camile and others to discuss their struggle with family separation.
- Discuss Camile's expectations of counseling.
- Encourage other therapists and interns to be culturally aware and to have high aspirations in particular for Students of Color.
- Engage in social justice efforts to improve equality for Black female students and access to student services.

ACCEPTING THE CHALLENGE

The challenge of becoming a culturally responsive therapist requires several assessment and related skill sets, as I have described. The treatment and prevention of psychosocial distress among Women of Color requires practitioners to use strategies that are based on culturally responsive, positive mental health proficiencies, practices, and paradigms that emphasize clients' strengths and recognize the deficits in the social, political, and economic systems (L. V. Jones & Warner, 2011). Feminist therapy is one such strategy. Women of Color's long history of mutual support, self-reliance, and participation in nonmainstream services (for example, religion, prayer, and community-based groups such as sororities) are consistent with the basic tenets of feminist theory and practice (L. S. Brown, 2018).

RECOMMENDATIONS FOR USE OF BLACK FEMINIST THERAPY

The appropriate use of Black feminist therapies with Women of Color requires literacy and competence on the part of practitioners, academics, and researchers, whether in the clinic, classroom, or institution. The following recommendations are suggested for therapists and allies interested in using the Black feminist perspective in mental health, education, and practice:

- Feminist therapists and their allies must have the courage to discuss and document their work on Black feminism in the practice literature and in public forums, such as at conferences, seminars, and other meetings on mental and social health. Therapists in academia should participate in continuing education programs that seek to enhance their practice skills and competency in the Black feminist perspective.
- Mental health practitioners must acknowledge their own value system and its potential impact on their ability to maintain an empathetic and therapeutic relationship with Women of Color in practice. Specifically, practitioners must be tuned in to diversity and its centrality to the ways in which their own values shape the therapeutic process.

- Mental health practitioners must possess the ability to recognize and the willingness to validate racism and the client's perceptions of the racism, discrimination, and bias that Women of Color have experienced in mental health and social service agencies, and they must provide a space in which Women of Color can share their identified problems without feeling invalidated or dismissed.

CONCLUSION

Effective services that aim to increase positive mental health outcomes for Women of Color's mental health challenges will influence policy, research, and practice decisions about future directions with this population. Mental health providers often face the challenge of documenting the extent of a social problem and developing interventions to eradicate it. It is clear that few data exist on the roles of gender, race, ethnicity, and culture in the epidemiology, assessment, and treatment of mental health disorders. As practitioners begin to apply strengths-based approaches, such as feminist therapy, with Women of Color, they will be able to assess the concepts' utility (L. V. Jones, 2004). Moreover, practitioners must recognize that, for interventions with Women of Color and their families to be successful, clients need accurate information and professional services that demonstrate respect and care for the person, the family, and the values and traditions they bring to the treatment process.

CHAPTER QUESTIONS

1. In what ways can mental health therapists demonstrate culturally competent and congruent practice?

2. What culturally congruent strategies can therapists include in the assessment process?

3. What micro-, mezzo-, and macro-level (institutional) changes are required at your agency to enhance cultural competence and culturally congruent therapy?

CHAPTER 4

Understanding Power and Powerlessness in Therapy with Women of Color

> *"Power wounding" invites clients (Women of Color), along with the clinician, to begin a dialogue to identify how the emotional injury occurred and what keeps it active, while also providing opportunities to imagine and take action on possibilities for healing.*
>
> —Vanessa Jackson (Pinderhughes et al., 2017, p. 58)

Power is a key concept in Black feminism, and it is essential to mental health treatment with many Women of Color. Unfortunately, powerlessness increases for many Women of Color as a result of their unrelenting exposure to intrusive, societally imposed oppression as well as their frequent struggle with the juxtaposition of pride and shame (L. V. Jones, 2017). These distinct oppressive challenges add a layer of complexity to some Women of Color's ability to function competently, and they often result in serious negative psychosocial consequences that are associated with powerlessness (for example, depression, anxiety, strained resources, poverty, poor health outcomes, exposure to violence, and drug addiction). In fact, it has been found that Women of Color experience disempowerment, which results in a sense of powerlessness, and are at high risk for developing mental health problems (Aiyer, Zimmerman, Morrel-Samuels, & Reischl, 2015; Ryan & Deci, 2000).

V. Jackson (2017) conceptualized Women of Color's sense of powerlessness as a "power wound" that can consist of an experience (emotional, physical, spiritual, financial, or sexual) and its aftermath that result in significant compromising of an individual's, community's, or society's ability to function, and specifically to take action, in their preferred manner. She posited that "the severity, intensity, or chronic nature of the wounding has a significant impact on the individual's or community's ability to function and heal" (p. 57). Hence, the exploration of power constrictions that result in a sense of powerlessness creates opportunities for Women of Color to reduce feelings of isolation and shame, which are common reactions when Women of Color are constricted by a narrow view of their problem. Unfortunately, traditional therapeutic approaches have overlooked the consequences of perceived and experienced powerlessness among many Women of Color in the United States (Wingo, 2001). Hence, a Black feminist lens in therapy provides an understanding of Women of Color's experiences of powerlessness, exposes the negative consequences of power dynamics on their psychosocial well-being, and allows the development of empowerment practices (Guy-Sheftall, 2005; V. Jackson, 2017). In this chapter, I contextualize power and powerlessness for Women of Color from an intersectional analysis, including how race, gender, and class interact with psychosocial stressors that trigger a cycle of powerlessness among Women of Color (L. V. Jones & Warner, 2011). Moreover, I discuss the lens of Black feminist praxis as a key construct for reclaiming power through self-empowerment and sociopolitical activism.

INTERSECTIONALITY AND WOMEN OF COLOR

Intersectionality, the study of the interactions of multiple systems of oppression or discrimination, has also been used as a tool for conceptualizing power among Women of Color (Symington, 2004). In recognizing the limitations of theorizing gender as a unified collective transcending race and class, intersectionality calls on scholars to be more inclusive of a broader group of women in their analysis of gender and definitions of what is feminist. In fact, intersectionality goes further to recognize that for many Women of Color, their feminist efforts are simultaneously embedded in and woven through their efforts against racism, classism, and other threats to their access to equal opportunities and social justice. More recently, intersectionality has proposed that gender cannot be used as a single analytic frame without also exploring how issues of race, sexuality, migration status, and social class affect one's experience as a woman (Guy-Sheftall, 2005). Consequently, scholars and theorists who endorse this theory must attend to myriad overlapping and mutually reinforcing oppressions that many women face in addition to gender. As previously discussed, it is no longer acceptable to produce analyses or theories of change that are embedded solely within a universal collective experience as "woman." Scholars such as Baca Zinn and Thornton Dill (1996), Collins (2000), and hooks (1981), among others, represent these efforts to dismantle theories of feminism and gender analyses that privilege a homogeneous portrayal of what is woman, womanist, feminine, or feminist. Use of the term "feminisms" in the plural to represent this diversity is an acknowledgment of these efforts.

Intersectionality calls on us to consider Women of Color as whole beings and to recognize that not all Women of Color experience their womanhood in the same ways. Many women face multiple forms of oppression, and not all women are rendered powerless. In fact, many Women of Color manage their multiple identities and challenges well and lead fulfilling lives. It is important to push this concept further and suggest that, individually, women experience various interlocking oppressions and a resulting sense of powerlessness differently (V. Jackson, 2017). Likewise, oppression in one context may be a privilege in another. This point challenges us to take a multisystemic approach to understanding power, powerlessness, and oppression within structural micro-interpersonal levels, as well as to understanding how these same social identities transcend more macro levels.

EXPLORING POWER AND POWERLESSNESS

Power, broadly defined, may entail the ability to bring about a desired effect on the micro (individual), mezzo (family, group), or macro (societal) level (McCubbin, 2001; Pinderhughes, 2017). In the context of psychological recovery, power can also be defined as having the opportunity to access valued materials and psychosocial resources that satisfy basic human needs, as well as to experience a level of competence that may instill a sense of stability and predictability in life (Prilleltensky, Nelson, & Peirson, 2001). Moreover, power can be expressed as an internal capacity to generate change and is often perceived as or manifested in one's sense of mastery or competence over self, environment, and others (Bruce & Thornton, 2004; Pinderhughes, 2017). Prilleltensky et al. (2001) defined power as the presence of opportunities to achieve outcomes. Although individuals can have power, it is not an individual characteristic; rather, it is relational in nature. Hence, Prilleltensky et al. noted that power lacks meaning when it is not in relationship to others or the environment, which links power to social, economic, political, and cultural occurrences. Negative forms of power, such as oppressive power, entail exploitation and exclusion based on differences. At the same time, protective and oppressive power is demonstrated as having power over someone, whereas cooperative power and collusive power lead to shared and collaborative forms of power. Caution is required in situations in which too much power can lead to misuse and abuse and when too little power can result in vulnerability and unmet needs (Prilleltensky et al., 2001).

While seeking to understand power relations among Women of Color, one may be abruptly confronted with grave misconceptions of identity, distortions of fact, and defensive attitudes. Historically and currently, most

Women of Color have been denied access to needed resources as a result of gender and racial oppression. This has made them susceptible to experiences of powerlessness, which, in turn, have placed them in unfavorable societal positions (S. A. Thomas & González-Prendes, 2009). *Powerlessness* is the inability to wield influence or gain needed resources such as income, education, and employment. For many Women of Color, powerlessness has restricted their ability to problem solve and increased their feelings of despair, vulnerability, low self-worth, and physical and emotional distress (Pinderhughes, 2017; S. A. Thomas & González-Prendes, 2009). Many Women of Color in subordinate positions present with powerlessness, sometimes expressed through behaviors that are perceived to be a sense of power. However, Women of Color who challenge or resist threats of powerlessness and annihilation in reaction to being overpowered are seen as being angry or uncooperative. Another common strategy often used by those who are powerless is to develop a self-perception that they are better than others by achieving competency or mastery in an area of their life such as education or their professional identity; others may display behaviors such as opposition, passive aggressiveness, manipulation, accommodation, and identification to turn their powerlessness into power. This exemplifies the cyclical nature of power and powerlessness in which individuals who feel powerless cope by developing power over others (Pinderhughes, 2017).

It has been easier to think of these behaviors as innate character flaws found in Women of Color. However, internalized rigid relational images such as these set everyone up to experience relational ruptures and disease. Looking at these phenomena through a Black feminist lens requires therapists to focus their attention on the systems that give rise to the individual behaviors and the individuals or groups who perpetuate those dysfunctional systems rather than on the individual herself. Powerlessness has a blunt and often complex effect on many Women of Color. The internal experience of powerlessness is related to an individual's belief that she has no control over the causes of or solutions to adverse life circumstances (Pinderhughes, 2017).

Many Women of Color in treatment display powerlessness when they attempt to manage economic, political, and social systems inherent in institutional oppression. Powerlessness implies that decision making is beyond the control of the individual, and it furthermore holds the person or system accountable for their lack of power. Powerlessness that is ongoing, consistent, and intractable plays a significant role in the mental and emotional dysfunction of Women of Color and often leads to negative coping responses (Hopps, Pinderhughes, & Shankar, 1995). Freeman (2008) discussed how some Women of Color react to their powerless positions by creating personalities that are contrary to societal norms and the values of the mainstream United States. This form of negative coping has led to poor decision-making skills that have criminalized Women of Color as a group. Pollack (2003) discussed how many imprisoned Women of Color turn to nonviolent crime and drugs, alcohol, or both in an effort to cope with life stressors and oppressive circumstances. As Michelle Alexander (2010) so eloquently shared in *The New Jim Crow: Mass Incarceration in the Age of Colorblindness*, U.S. society would rather portray Women of Color as criminals, unemployed, or single parents on welfare than place them in the context of their oppressive life experiences.

A comprehensive understanding of factors associated with powerlessness and psychosocial stressors among Women of Color remains elusive. However, researchers have identified that oppressive social conditions such as institutional and ethnocentric practices are related to the development of mental health disorders among Women of Color (Grote, Bledsoe, Larkin, Lemay, & Brown, 2007). In particular, stress (Grote, Bledsoe, Larkin, et al., 2007); negative thinking patterns (Delahanty et al., 2001); and institutional racism, sexism, and other experiences of discrimination have been linked to depression among Women of Color. In addition, research on the impact of stress on adverse health outcomes among Women of Color is growing (L. V. Jones, 2017). According to Geronimus et al. (2007), the psychological and physiological responses to stress experienced by many Women of Color over the life course lead to chronic physical and psychological health problems. Studies reviewed by Thomas and González-Prendes (2009) showed a range of health problems created or exacerbated among Women of Color by their association with anger and stress related to powerlessness. Consequently, an important goal of therapists is to reduce stress in an effort to promote positive health and mental health outcomes among Women of Color.

The question of how to address powerlessness is often asked, especially when considering this issue with people of privilege and those in controlling positions. The importance of acknowledging a privilege viewpoint becomes a part of this question. Differences in power are less apparent to people in privileged positions because people in privileged situations are more willing to accept a view of U.S. society as classless and colorblind, supporting what the literature has described as the myth of the level playing field. However, this viewpoint ignores the experience of marginalized groups and people in less privileged positions, and it discounts issues such as discrimination and injustice that these groups frequently face. The social differences can become extremely relevant to some while remaining obscured to those who view the world as equal.

When power differences are not addressed, the disconnect between oppressed and privileged groups likely remains (Browne & Mills, 2001; Proctor, 2008). Through educational and training opportunities, along with experience, people may begin to recognize and acknowledge their cultural biases. Acknowledgment of cultural biases leads people to become more aware of their endorsement of Eurocentric attitudes and behaviors. These attitudes and behaviors could be represented in styles of communication, nonverbal behaviors, and beliefs and values about society, family, and individuals. A deconstructive examination of one's own views can help one to move beyond a one-sided description, such as a "them" and "us" viewpoint, and more toward a dialogue in which one's cultural assumptions are questioned (Proctor, 2008).

EMPOWERMENT AS CENTRAL TO THERAPEUTIC WORK WITH WOMEN OF COLOR

Therapists have traditionally been viewed as expert helpers who diagnose, teach, and treat, whereas the client is seen as the one seeking assistance with his or her need. Therapeutic relationships often expose Women of Color to double vulnerability by compounding the power differentials that exist between therapist and client, as well as their respective cultural identity (Pinderhughes, 2017). Therapists may use their power over minority clients, including Women of Color, to satisfy personal needs for power and recognition by viewing their clients as incompetent, thus bolstering their own sense of competence (Glover, 2003). Powerlessness among Women of Color can be decreased in the therapist–client relationship when the decision-making process is collaborative and shared. Grant and Cadell (2009) discussed the circular relationship of knowledge and power in that knowledge generates and sustains power, and power creates and sustains knowledge. Therapists must become aware of the effect their knowledge and experience may have on clients. In particular, power relations cannot be ignored with Women of Color because therapists may have to forfeit their feelings of expertise to empower these women. This vigilance is necessary to guard against the clinician's normal vulnerability to reinforce powerlessness in their work with Women of Color. For instance, the helping relationship should be one of collaboration, trust, and shared power so that the therapist does not replicate the feelings of powerlessness (Gutierrez, 1990). The sharing of power creates a freedom from dominance in which the sense of conflict, fear, stress, and rigidity and the need for sameness are relinquished. Likewise, the freedom from the loss of power, the pressure to hold on to it, irrational thinking, and the intolerance of difference is unleashed (Glover, 2003; Pinderhughes, 2017).

Empowerment perspectives assume that the roles of power and powerlessness are integral to the mental health treatment experiences of Women of Color (Gutierrez, 1990). According to Browne and Mills (2001), *empowerment* is "the gaining of power by an individual, family group, or community" (p. 23). Empowerment assumes a position of powerlessness on the part of the client group. The process of empowerment has been used to help populations of disenfranchised people rise above situations as well as foster strength in individuals who experience feelings of powerlessness (Tew, 2006). People who occupy powerless roles in more than one area of their life can perceive empowerment as double victimization, and the process of empowerment may require targeted or expanded strategies (Pinderhughes, 1989). "Double victims" may have to work twice as hard to develop coping strategies, but if one powerless role is linked with another powerless role, it is possible that modifications to one role may facilitate alterations in another (Glover, 2003; Gutierrez, 1990). Hence, empowerment is the process of increasing personal, interpersonal, and political power so that people are motivated and encouraged to improve their overall well-being. In developing empowerment-based, culturally relevant interventions grounded in Black feminisms, methods must be structured in a manner in which Women of Color can experience themselves as competent in the context of a supportive environment (L. V. Jones, 2004). Empowerment techniques that enable people to experience themselves as competent, valuable, and worthwhile, both as an individual in society and as a member of a cultural group, help create a sense of control in people's lives. Effective empowerment strategies may require therapists to become vulnerable by using strategies that eschew power derived from their position as expert or from a particular cultural group and avoiding stereotypes (L. V, Jones, 2009).

Knowledge of empowerment strategies that enhance one's psychosocial competence provides a foundation on which a student or professional might begin to think about interventions for this population. For example, empowerment-based perspectives draw on psychosocial competence rather than pathological or maladaptive behaviors (L. V. Jones & Warner, 2011). Thus, interventions in the mental health field should aim to help Women of Color sort out the personal from the contextual by helping them recognize how the internalization of socially constructed identities has contributed to their depressive symptoms (C. B. Williams, 2005).

RECLAIMING POWER: WOMEN OF COLOR'S ENGAGEMENT IN ACTIVISM

Activism has become an essential part of Black feminist praxis and, as such, seeks to empower the individual and increase the interpersonal and political power of oppressed and marginalized populations for individual and collective transformation (Gutierrez, 1990; Lee, 2001). Black feminist activism helps Women of Color to understand how they are oppressed and dominated, and it often inspires them to engage in efforts to bring about broader social change. Moreover, Black feminist activism often requires the rejection of traditional gender expectations and the recognition of sexist power imbalances in society (Guy-Sheftall, 2005). Central to Black feminist activism is the belief that the inferior status delegated to women is due to societal inequality; that the personal status of women is shaped by political, economic, and social power relations; and that women should have equal access to all forms of power.

Many community and Black feminist scholar activists have challenged sexist forms of oppression through many means, including confronting exploitation, harassment, and objectification (Staggenborg & Taylor, 2005). Although some of these resistances and challenges to patriarchy occur on the individual level, feminists can also challenge existing power structures and norms through collective resistance. Black feminist social movements have ushered in some major changes in the United States toward the reclamation of power (A. Jones, Eubanks, & Smith, 2014). Community-organizing traditions that have been practiced and refined for decades by Women of Color such as Sojourner Truth, Fannie Lou Hamer, Ella Baker, and Marsha P. Johnson have empowered new generations of Women of Color to demand that their experiences be made central to community concerns.

Women of Color who joined consciousness-raising groups in the 1960s and 1970s began to connect with other women, and in sharing their experiences they learned to see the political nature of their personal problems (Carr, 2003). Feminist views can restore individuals' sense of personal power, strength, and capacity to handle life's problems (Handy & Kassam, 2006). Specifically, Women of Color and their allies create massive feminist movements that collectively challenge the structural sources of male privilege. The Combahee River Collective (CRC), founded in Boston by three self-identified queer Women of Color feminists, Demita Frazier, Beverly Smith, and Barbara Smith, issued one of the clearest and most effective documents on the intersections of racial, gender, and sexual oppression. They have also recently been credited with articulating the true inclusive power of identity politics. "Most radical politics come directly" from Women of Color's identity, the women wrote in the CRC Statement (CRC, 1986). "If Black women were free, it would mean that everyone else would have to be free since our freedom would necessitate the destruction of all the systems of oppression" CRC, 1986, p. 15). These movements have provided a platform on which accessible dialogue can occur between Women of Color and the larger public regarding their multiplicative oppressive injustices.

At the same time, Women of Color have been leading some of the most vibrant protests of the past few years, such as Black Lives Matter (BLM), the Standing Rock pipeline protests, and the Dreamers movement. In these movements, gender and sexuality are framed as integral to the issues of racism, immigration, and environmental protection. These movements are an integral part of a "new women's movement," and they point out the importance of defining that movement broadly. Examples are the #MuteRKelly movement, Women's March, BLM, and the #MeToo movement. These campaigns have challenged institutional forms of privilege, oppression, sexual exploitation, and patriarchy. Although one of the main goals of BLM is to fight against systematic violence by police and private citizens against People of Color in the United States, another one of its objectives is to reform Black activism. BLM's organizational founders, and other members of the larger Movement for Black Lives collective, have insisted on discourses of intersectionality that value and center all Black lives, including, among others, Women of Color, femmes, and queer and trans folk. This stands in contrast to the impulses of the historical People of Color freedom movement, which chose to center cisgender Black men in racial justice struggles, intentionally and strategically marginalizing cisgender Black women and queer folks who might be seen as unworthy of rights within the logics of capitalist heteropatriarchy (A. Jones, Eubanks, & Smith, 2014).

The goals of BLM are to encourage empathy for Black communities, illustrate lingering institutional oppression, and work toward policy changes that make everyone safer, all while shifting Black activism's history of elevating straight men over Black women. Along with other BLM founders Opal Tometi and Patrisse Cullors, Alicia Garza has long insisted on the radical intersectionality of the phrase, writing,

> Black Lives Matter is a unique contribution that goes beyond extrajudicial killings of Black people by police and vigilantes. It goes beyond the narrow nationalism that can be prevalent within some Black communities, which merely call on Black people to love Black, live Black and buy Black, keeping straight cis Black men in the front of the movement while our sisters, queer and trans and disabled folk, take up roles in the background or not at all. Black Lives Matter affirms the lives of Black queer and trans folks, disabled folks, Black-undocumented folks, folks with records, women and all Black lives along the gender spectrum. (Garza, 2014, pp. 1–3)

We can also examine the activism of the Black Women's Blueprint, who established the Black Women's Truth and Reconciliation Commission. The Black Women's Truth and Reconciliation Commission focuses on sexual violence against Black women in the United States as a human rights atrocity. This movement was organized by women and girls of African descent (many of whom were denied access to and assistance from the criminal justice system) to encourage engagement in collective transformation regarding injustices and harms they experienced. In these examples, Women of Color found it necessary to have solidarity around the fact of race, gender, class, and all other forms of oppression. Hence, Black feminist activism may differ from other forms of feminist activism in that it not only centers on the struggles and empowerment of Women of Color, but also provides a theoretical framework to unveil matrices of intersectionality.

CONCLUSION

Effective services that are aimed at increasing positive mental health outcomes for Women of Color experiencing societally imposed oppression should be an item of high importance to therapists. Given its potential applicability to Women of Color in therapy, the Black feminist paradigm offers a unique opportunity to work toward these goals. It also offers practitioners a useful method of providing services from an empowerment-based perspective. This method differs from traditional medical models used in treating stress and other related mental health disorders among Women of Color.

At the micro level, empowerment in Black feminism is the mobilization of the client's uniqueness and self-determination to take charge of her own life, to learn new ways of thinking about the problem situation, and to adopt new behaviors that reflect positive outcomes. Mental health therapists are often given the challenge of documenting the extent of a social problem and developing interventions to eradicate it. As I have highlighted here, it is clear that few data exist on the role of gender, race, ethnicity, and culture in disorders and interventions, as well as in the epidemiology, assessment, and treatment of mental health stressors. As therapists begin to apply empowerment-based concepts, such as psychosocial competence, with Women of Color, they will be able to assess the concepts' utility (L. V. Jones, 2017). Moreover, therapists must recognize that for interventions with Women of Color and their families to be successful, clients need accurate information and professional services that demonstrate respect and care for the person, family, values, and traditions that they bring to the treatment process. Practitioners must also ascertain whether members of a woman's microsystem, such as family members, friends, and small groups, can be linked to the roots of the problem.

At the macro level, there is a need to recognize potential links between problems and environmental factors. Macro-level empowerment recognizes the need for large-scale organizational and institutional change. Group empowerment involves the ability to work with others to change social institutions. For example, the absence of ethnic-specific community organizations that offer culturally responsive treatment services can contribute to Women of Color's sense of isolation and alienation. Because it allows for a thorough analysis of multiple interactions between the micro and macro contexts, the psychosocial competence framework is an important tool for policy and research that focus on addressing issues of importance to Women of Color. Examining both micro and macro contexts allows for the development of policies and research that focus on specific and larger societal barriers to treatment of mental health issues among Women of Color.

Black feminism emphasizes the social, political, and economic structures that shape human societies and stresses that gender must be considered when examining the effects of oppression, domination, power, and powerlessness in the lives of Women of Color. Black feminist therapists, scholars, and activists must encourage women in therapy to reclaim power to the extent possible in our society through political and social activism. Therapists fighting for sexual and reproductive rights, access to affordable child care, and equal pay for equal work must also work collectively to address powerlessness and domination among Women of Color and other marginalized or oppressed populations.

CHAPTER QUESTIONS

1. Discuss your experiences with power wounds, whether emotional, physical, spiritual, financial, or sexual.
2. In an effort to overcome a sense of powerlessness, have you ever "power wounded" someone else?
3. How might Women of Color experience power imbalances similarly to and differently from themselves?
4. What steps should practitioners take to heal from power wounds and empower Women of Color?

CHAPTER 5

Applying Black Feminist Therapy Approaches to Women of Color in Therapy

Are you sure, sweetheart, that you want to be well?

—Toni Cade Bambara (1980, p. 3), *The Salt Eaters*

As a Black feminist therapist, I am often absorbed by the recurrent question of healing and wellness offered to Women of Color in Toni Cade Bambara's 1980 novel *The Salt Eaters:* "Are you sure, sweetheart, that you want to be well? . . . Just so's you're sure, sweetheart, and ready to be healed, cause wholeness is no trifling matter. A lot of weight when you're well" (p. 3). In this novel, Cade Bambara's intent is neither to induce revolution nor to offer readers her vision of political and social change. Instead, she prepares her readers, in particular Women of Color, for the difficult healing work along their life journeys.

In Black feminist therapy, this rhetorical question can be posed to Women of Color and to therapists to encourage them to use frameworks that resist socially imposed definitions of success that do not reflect the values, coping mechanisms, emotional support systems, or general reality of Women of Color. There is an opportunity to validate and use Women of Color's traditional methods of coping and healing, such as reliance on family, use of nontraditional healers, prayer, racial pride, spirituality, religion, community connectedness, and resourcefulness. The absence of knowledge regarding Women of Color's native coping skills leaves a gap in the development of appropriate interventions. To support the emotional healing and wellness of Women of Color, therapists of all races should embrace psychological frameworks, such as the Black feminist framework, that assist in their liberation from experienced oppressions (for example, racism, sexism, heterosexism, classism, ageism) and from internalized oppression (the effects of historical oppression, passed on from one generation to the next).

Black feminist therapeutic spaces have been identified as radical therapeutic spaces in which Women of Color can share their challenges and expand their empowerment and sense of joy in their lives. Black feminist therapy recognizes and explores intersections of identity and Women of Color's resulting life circumstances, both good and bad (that is, the way in which gender, race, sexual orientation, religion, nationality, and a host of other identity markers shape their experience in and of the world). Through this process, Women of Color come to understand how their personality and coping styles evolved, and they learn how to break free from damaging patterns and from mainstream White, middle-class social and cultural expectations that Women of Color internalize, especially with regard to race, gender, class, and sexual orientation. Black feminist therapy combines consciousness-raising (understanding of one's race and gender roles), empowerment tactics, self-exploration, and relationships and joy and makes healing and growth possible in therapy. In Black feminist healing spaces, Women of Color can tell their stories and be heard by an understanding and nonjudgmental therapist who understands their history of struggle and their current challenges of living in a racist and sexist society. Their experiences, pain, struggles, and achievements are wholly witnessed in Black feminist therapy, which helps them to better re-examine their experiences and feelings and achieve their goals. In this way, they can reassess and reconfigure these experiences, often shifting the blame, guilt, and shame from themselves to the sexist and racist social forces that helped to create these experiences, and recover from psychosocial traumas, ultimately creating strategies for change.

WHY WOMEN OF COLOR SEEK TREATMENT

Women of Color pursue therapy for a myriad of reasons. Some seek treatment to cope with major life changes, such as race and sexual identity questioning, underemployment, workplace or academic stress related to racism, or interracial coupling conflicts. Others may seek help to address chronic stress, depression, toxic levels of racism and sexism, feelings of isolation or alienation from community, eating disorders, drug- and alcohol-related problems, or intergenerational traumatic family patterns that they have unwittingly embraced. Many identify specific issues or goals that they want to work on in therapy; others seek therapy after family, friends, clergy, or medical professionals suggest that they do so to help them cope with ongoing problems (Boyd-Franklin, 2006). Whatever the motivation, we must acknowledge their courage to ask for help, show up, and stand ready to do the work. This acknowledgment is especially helpful given the negative perception of seeking professional help in Communities of Color, where many believe that therapy is an indulgence, a type of coddling and privilege in which White, middle-class, or wealthy women engage.

These women often enter therapy with descriptions of themselves and an understanding of their problems in stereotypically racist and classist terms. Part of the ongoing struggle in the context of mental health therapy is to boldly challenge their sense of self or their individually or societally overdetermined identity. One would think that people would be eager to give up this degraded sense of self, but often they are not, partly because doing so requires coming to terms with the fact that they, their children, and their families are poor and that this is a social–historical fact rather than a personal flaw.

Issues related to motherhood also emerge in the treatment of poor Women of Color. They often express guilt over how they attempt to protect their children from poverty or spend their lives trying to make up to them for its existence. See, for instance, the case of an African American young woman, Crystal:

> Crystal had a baby at age 14 by Steve, her 15-year-old boyfriend. Both Crystal and Steve grew up in a rural section of New Jersey in very poor families and communities. Crystal's mother was angry about the pregnancy, noting, "I can't feed and clothe you and your siblings. We don't need another body in this house." Because of her religious beliefs, her mother insisted that Crystal could not have an abortion. As Crystal progressed in her pregnancy, she and her mother were called in by the school. School administrators informed them that the school could not meet her needs as a pregnant student, especially given that she had missed several days during the first trimester of her pregnancy, and the school administrators suggested she withdraw until the following school year. Crystal's mother grew more frustrated and disappointed with Crystal and insisted that "giving up this child is the only option." Steve disappeared sometime during the later months of the pregnancy, and his mother denied that Crystal was pregnant by her son. Crystal did her best to ignore the fact that she was pregnant. Hating every moment of it, she neglected her health and the health of the baby by not engaging in prenatal care. She eventually had a healthy baby girl, and after giving birth, she gave her baby over to child welfare. She escaped to upstate New York, where she constantly obsessed over her "failure" to be a good mother (a societal failure), and for the next three years, she suffered through a nervous breakdown. After hospitalization for a suicide attempt, Crystal was referred for mental health treatment.

Crystal's story exemplifies the view that poverty is a personal affliction rather than a failure of society to create opportunities for all of its members to live worthwhile lives. Many poor women have at some point been forced to make use of the foster care system or fallen under the scrutiny of the Bureau of Child Welfare; more often than not, this has resulted in their being labeled unfit, abusive, or both. The destructiveness of such labels is twofold: first, the social stigma of being identified as unfit; second, the absence of support provided to the mother. These labels in no way enhance the likelihood of positively changing the relationship between mothers and their children. If anything, it increases the shame, humiliation, and anger that these mothers experience.

This syndrome of shame, blame, and abuse has been identified in the therapeutic field, and therapists now recognize the tendency of these women to try to make up to their children for being poor and unfit and for the abuse that their children heap on them beginning at very early ages. This abuse serves as a way for the young people to cover up and not come to terms with who they are and the constraints and limitations that class and race have inflicted on them. The overwhelming message to their mother is "You owe me." It is yet another way in which new generations are taught the sexism that is pervasive in this society.

Several themes appear with some frequency in the mental health literature on Women of Color's psychotherapeutic needs and reasons for seeking therapy: racial isolation, sexual trauma, stress from being a caregiver to multiple family and community members, internalized oppression, and the need to integrate multiple identities (for example, mother, wife, caretaker, Black woman) (Constantine, 2002; Harley, Jolivette, McCormick, & Tice, 2002; S. J. Jones, 2003; C. B. Williams, 2005). Nonetheless, there are salient issues that therapists would be wise to look and listen for that are likely to affect the therapeutic relationship between the client and her therapist. Specifically, I focus on issues of identity and self-esteem, resilience, and vulnerability, as well as attachment and dependency. I believe that these developmental issues are affected by cultural norms as well as by sexism and racism in the larger society. Therapists must also be aware of the triple jeopardy Women of Color experience by virtue of their membership in multiple devalued groups (Guy-Sheftall 1995). Specifically, racism, sexism, and classism—the legacy of slavery—continue to the present day (hooks, 1981; L. C. Jackson & Greene, 2000). This "triple whammy" has an impact on Women of Color's identity and self-esteem. Thus, identity development and the development of a positive sense of self are affected by the internalization of racial and gender stereotypes, as well as by the experience of external racial or gender trauma. In addition, classism negatively affects psychological well-being while serving as a hindrance to upward mobility for Women of Color seeking to escape poverty (American Psychological Association, 2019). Often, Women of Color's struggles with identity and self-esteem are manifested in concerns about looks and beauty (Okazawa-Rey, Robinson & Ward, 1987). Reid (1988) pointed out that Women of Color represent the antithesis of what is considered American female beauty. In terms of skin color, hair texture and length, facial features, and body shape, most Women of Color do not approach the European American ideal of beauty.

THREE THEMES IN CLINICAL PRACTICE

Three themes have consistently arisen in clinical practice with Women of Color: the inability to recognize and own that they have been victims, sexual devaluation and victimization, and reliance on the Strong Black Woman (SBW) persona and how to replace it.

Inability to Admit to Being a Victim

Women of Color often enter therapy in an effort to make sense of subtle yet toxic racist and sexist microaggressions they have experienced in the past and the present. I first present the academic definition of a microaggression and then translate it into a term readily understood by Women of Color, as a "dardo psicológico," or psychological dart (L. V. Jones, Ahn, Quezada, & Chakravarty, 2018). *Microaggression* refers to ordinary verbal, nonverbal, and environmental insults, slurs, or abuses, "whether intentional or unintentional, which communicate hostile, derogatory, or negative messages" (D. W. Sue et al., 2007, p. 273) to Women of Color solely on the basis of their marginalized status as Women of Color. In many cases, these hidden messages invalidate, denigrate, threaten, and intimidate Women of Color and make them feel as though they do not belong with the majority group (D. W. Sue, Capodilupo, & Holder, 2008). For instance, many Women of Color in the workforce are continually challenged about their knowledge and credentials and forced to prove their competency; they constantly have to validate their ideas, decisions, judgments, and expertise to gain credibility with colleagues. Moreover, psychological darts or microaggressions serve as daily reminders that one's race, ethnicity, and gender are ongoing triggers in the world (Harrell, 2000). The demeaning nature of experiencing a wounding microaggression or psychological dart can make women feel marginalized and affect their self-esteem (Harrell, 2000). In a discussion of the meaning of psychological darts, a middle-age Black woman who is currently working on her PhD in engineering pointedly shared,

> Psychological darts, they are real. . . . They are sometimes visible or invisible weapons used against us [women of African descent], through mental warfare. . . . They say, "You sound so eloquent," "I didn't know you were so smart," "How'd you get an A?" "I thought you were a secretary in the department when I first met you."

She further stated, "I often feel as if I'm wounded over and over again. The bad thing is that you can't armor yourself, because you don't know when it will happen again."

For decades, parents of color have told their children that to succeed despite racial discrimination, they need to be "twice as good": twice as smart, twice as dependable, twice as talented. This advice can be found in everything from literature to television shows to day-to-day conversation.

The cumulative impact of surviving these psychological darts can harm the overall health of Women of Color (Utsey, Ponterotto, Reynolds, & Cancelli, 2000). One study (Clark, Anderson, Clark, & Williams, 1999) framed the impact of racism on Women of Color in a contextual model, suggesting that a race- or gender-based encounter—when perceived as racist or sexist—acts as a stressor that elicits coping responses as well as psychological and physiological stress responses, which can, in turn, lead to negative health outcomes. Comas-Díaz and Jacobsen (2001) further posited that some Women of Color may sustain lasting psychological injury from traumatic racial victimization, which results in hypervigilance and hypersensitivity to potential racial victimization in ambiguous social situations. In addition, these experiences may be associated with depression, anxiety, lower well-being, lower self-regard, and ill health (Donovan, Galban, Grace, Bennett, & Felicié, 2012; D. W. Sue et al., 2007).

Unfortunately, many Women of Color often underreport mental health symptoms because they tend to internalize these experiences as a fact of life or they do not see them as problematic enough to report (Neal-Barnett & Crowther, 2000). Women of Color often normalize or internalize such psychic injuries in an effort to survive emotionally, socially, and physically. Black feminist therapists, or therapists aiming to work more effectively with Women of Color, must recognize that Women of Color may have difficulty identifying feelings such as anger, shame, and low self-esteem, as well as the sources of these feelings, because of their tendency to normalize racist and sexist microaggressions.

Sexual Devaluation and Victimization

All women, regardless of race or ethnicity, are at risk for sexual victimization, including the aforementioned microaggressions, along with childhood sexual abuse, rape, and the range of sexual harassment. However, Women of Color are at greater risk of experiencing sexual victimization over the course of their lifetime (Giscombe, 2018). For instance, a study by Wyatt (1992) involving a community sample of women found that Women of Color experienced a higher proportion of attempted sexual assault (27 percent) than White women (17 percent) and that Women of Color reported a higher rate of incest survival. Russell, Schurman, and Trocki (1988) further reported that, compared with White women, Women of Color experience more severe victimization, greater traumatic long-term effects, and more adverse life experiences as a result of their abuse.

Unfortunately, society (that is, White, patriarchal, and middle-class social norms) socializes Women of Color to believe from a young age that they are at high risk for victimization, objectification, and rape rather than teaching them that they are valued and worthy of living violence free. Despite the current national attention to movements such as #MeToo and #MuteRKelly, Women of Color continue to have a history of being demeaned and denigrated through messages about their sexuality, which affect not only how they see themselves, but also how they develop relationships with others. The perpetuation of stereotypic images of Women of Color, such as the Jezebel (sexy woman), reinforces and serves to justify sexual exploitation (Greene, 1994). The lack of credibility afforded Women of Color may explain why they are more likely than White women to wait before revealing their sexual assault (64 percent versus 36 percent, respectively). Moreover, failure to receive a supportive response from family members, police officials, and health care providers may reinforce feelings of shame and contribute to hesitancy to reveal victimization in the future (Wyatt, 1992).

In some ways, devaluation is more straightforward for Women of Color than denial. Devaluation holds that the things Women of Color report about their traumas are actually not as important as the victims imagine them to be. Denial can create a facade that once the victims come forward with better proof of their accusations, the public (for example, institutions of justice, health agencies, family, friends) will be enraged. In contrast, devaluation conveys that even if sexually victimized Women of Color can prove beyond a shadow of a doubt that something happened exactly as they claim it did, the public will simply minimize the seriousness of what occurred, refusing to classify what happened as an injustice. Either there was no injustice because the claimed brutality did not take place (denial), or there was no injustice because the brutality that plainly did take place is tolerable (devaluation). This is seen in the story of Lynn:

> Lynn was raped at 16 by an upstanding man in the community. He had been extremely kind to Lynn, and one afternoon she accompanied him to a hotel to pick up some of his things. When she realized that his intentions were sexual, she said no. He raped her. Her mother learned of the incident but decided not to do anything about it, not even talking to Lynn (denial). Lynn confronted her rapist, and he said, "You know you wanted it." Lynn became very depressed and anxious but understood she needed to reach out for help. She is in therapy, but her family continues to understand her rape as her fault because at the age 16 "she had no business going to that hotel"; therefore, they do not affirm the injustice that Lynn is experiencing (devaluation).

The narratives of systemic oppressive aggressions and macroaggressions committed against Women of Color continue to create a culture of devaluation and promote negative stereotypes of Women of Color. Such widespread and culturally accepted negative sexual stereotypes have a grave impact on the way they—including the younger generation, who have had more consciousness-raising—view themselves and negotiate their social interactions and their sexual experiences. With frequent exposure to negative sexual stereotypes, many Women of Color come to therapy with internalized negative images of themselves, low self-esteem, or negative cognitive sexual schemas based on those images (Stephens & Few, 2007). Diagnostically, these women present with characteristics of depression, drug abuse, suicidal ideation, eating disorders, and somatic complaints. Moreover, Women of Color who have internalized oppression or who have experienced rape, incest, emotional or physical abuse, or a negative backlash from their partners, family members, or friends may feel less in control of their bodies and the sexual decisions that they make (for example, body shaming, unprotected sex, multiple partners). As a result, they are at high risk for unwanted pregnancy and sexually transmitted diseases (STDs), including HIV/AIDS.

For instance, a client shared that she was molested at age 12 years but "thought nothing of it. Actually, I always thought it just happened." In a later session, I discussed how nonchalant she was about sharing her experience, as though she was to be held accountable for someone else's actions: "Reflecting on your current battle with anxiety, I'm wondering how much your past trauma is showing up in your current illness." She responded, "I have to live in denial; no one else cared then [35 years ago], and no one cares now. My ex-husband [who was of Asian descent] said, 'You Black women are always looking for it, or blaming your actions on others.'" She continued, "I've been devastated and outraged my whole life, but it's best if I keep it to myself."

As this example illustrates, what makes the experience of devaluation and victimization even more problematic is the tendency for Women of Color to blame themselves and remain silent about their experiences and their emotional impact. This silence can stem from their oppression and abuse, and being able to voice their feelings and describe their experiences to an understanding and nonjudgmental counselor offers Women of Color an avenue through which to process their feelings, move toward recovery, and assert their feelings and desires in the future, avoiding their vulnerability to further abuse and oppression. Therapy is particularly useful for Women of Color when they do not have community support to help them to gain agency and power in interpersonal relationships.

Consequently, race, socioeconomic class, and cultural images internalized by both the client and the therapist must be examined in the therapeutic relationship, particularly when assessing mental health disorders among

Black women (B. W. Thompson, 1992). Therapists must be prepared to address these concerns by raising such questions as "What messages and values did you receive from family, peers, your community, and the larger society about valued physical features and regarding beauty such as body size, weight, skin color, facial features, and hair?" and "What messages did your family, teachers, and the larger society give you about life chances and career choices based on education, intelligence, and beauty?" Insight and therapeutic progress can be made by breaking the silence around these internalized, often stifling messages (Greene, 1994). Awareness of the internalized negative self-images of one's sexual self and the degree to which a client adopts this image can provide some additional insight when conducting an assessment and therapy with the sexually victimized Women of Color.

Black feminist therapists working with Women of Color must be prepared to go beyond traditional approaches that attribute sexual problems to intrapsychic difficulties, faulty learning, or both. This can be better understood by conducting a nonjudgmental historical discussion of these negative self-images as well as the implications of adhering to them. It is important to explore how these self-images affect their self-esteem, intimate relationships, and sexual behavior (for example, choosing inappropriate partners, not taking adequate precautions to avoid STDs, unwanted pregnancy). In cases in which a woman tries to counter the image of Women of Color as hypersexualized or Jezebels by avoiding sexual intercourse, it may be necessary to conduct some basic sex education to reduce misinformation. Sexual assertiveness skills, such as discussing sexual needs with partners and identifying techniques for initiating and engaging in sexual intercourse, can also be beneficial. Last, initiating a discussion of sexual violence in a safe therapeutic environment and dispelling the myth that Women of Color somehow deserve to be victims of sexual violence may reduce the level of shame and hesitancy to reveal and discuss their victimization. Therapists must be fully committed to not canceling out Women of Color's experiences or their struggles.

Reliance on the SBW Ideology

The SBW stereotype views Women of Color as victims of the toxic patriarchal society in which they are driven to fit the standard mold of a traditional SBW (Beauboeuf-Lafontant, 2009; Woods-Giscombé, 2010). This ideological mythology exists for women throughout the African diaspora and for descendants of the Spanish and Portuguese colonization. Women of Color must manage multiple roles as mother, grandmother, employee, wife, and caretaker to their extended family and community (Donovan & West, 2014; Romero, 2000). As posited by numerous scholars (Beauboeuf-Lafontant, 2009; Romero, 2000; C. B. Williams, 2005; Woods-Giscombé, 2010), the SBW ideology is rooted in slavery: Being strong and caring for children, extended family, and community began as a survival response to an existence laden with violence, exploitation, rape, and oppression. Today, the SBW lens persists in that the broader society views Women of Color as naturally resilient, self-sacrificing, and able to handle, with ease, the myriad stressors and traumas life throws at them (C. B. Williams, 2005). Moreover, Women of Color are viewed as self-reliant and emotionally contained (Harrington, Crowther, & Shipherd, 2010; Romero, 2000). They nurture by providing emotional, spiritual, and financial support (Beauboeuf-Lafontant, 2009; Harrington et al., 2010; Romero, 2000). Regarding caregiving, the SBW is perceived as self-sacrificing, putting everyone else's needs before her own (Beauboeuf-Lafontant, 2009; Harrington et al., 2010; Romero, 2000). In the community, she is sought out because of her perceived wisdom and her generous offering of her time, energy, and resources to those who need them without resentment or expectation of reciprocation (Beauboeuf-Lafontant, 2009; Harrington et al., 2010; Romero, 2000). Her strength is also shown in her independence, self-control, and strong work ethic (Woods-Giscombé, 2010).

Research has suggested that many Women of Color may have internalized the SBW ideology as a way to cope with multiple oppressive forces such as racism, sexism, and classism (Donovan & West, 2014). Studies have revealed that high internalization of the SBW ideology may be linked directly or indirectly to such negative outcomes as depression, overeating, self-silencing, and reduced help seeking and self-care (Donovan & West, 2014; Harrington et al., 2010; Woods-Giscombé, 2010). Some of the main tenets of the SBW image—namely, self-reliance and emotional containment—however, have also been found to exacerbate the negative outcomes of stress (Romero, 2000; Woods-Giscombé, 2010). Whereas this myth may be seen as helpful in some ways, the internalization of SBW ideology may have a negative impact on women's health if they believe that they do not need to seek help; if they believe that they can get through distress, addictions, a violent past, and so forth by coping on their own; or if they use it as a mechanism to cope with their depression and stress. Many Women of Color clients reveal that buying into the SBW image has limited their ability to seek help or express negative emotions such as sadness, anger, or frustration.

For example, in a qualitative study that investigated Women of Color's responses to depression, Nicolaidis et al. (2010) found that the SBW image acted as a barrier to acknowledging depressive symptoms, accepting a diagnosis, and help seeking. Romero (2000) further posited that Women of Color who identify with the image of the SBW have difficulty starting and staying in therapy because of their ambivalence toward acknowledging the need for help and focusing on self-care. Understanding how Black women perceive and internalize the SBW image is important not only for therapists to support Black women in reducing their anxiety and depression, but also to alleviate health conditions such as hypertension and obesity (Flegal, Carroll, Ogden, & Curtin, 2010; Neal-Barnett, 2003; Rosenthal & Schreiner, 2000). Therapists providing Black feminist therapy or working with Girls and Women of Color can launch discussions that aim to redefine strength and what it means to be strong, Black or Brown, and female. For example, it is possible to change Women of Color's cognitive contingencies of "If I'm not independent, then I am weak or an imposter" to "If I ask for support, then I am recognizing my strength and my value." By using a Black feminist lens, therapists can help Women of Color redefine what strength means and acknowledge a true and more authentic version of themselves.

THERAPEUTIC CONSIDERATIONS

In this chapter, I provide several general considerations for therapy with Black women. It is crucial that therapists working with Women of Color understand and empathize with societal constructs of culturally imposed images, such as the SBW or the sexy Jezebel. These images may influence Black women quite differently than myths or ideals influence women of other racial groups. As a way to become more aware of these influences, therapists can engage in both didactic and experiential training, and they can use professional resources to better understand these images (for example, Goings, 1994; Turner, 1994). Therapists can also increase their own awareness by being more sensitive to how Black women are portrayed in the media, magazines, and other public communication forums. Engaging in informed, explicit discussions with clients regarding the impact of such images on their self-image and self-esteem is also important and can communicate a sense of respect for the client's racial and cultural background. These education and awareness efforts help to foster a greater sensitivity to cultural and racial influences and can result in a more comprehensive and enlightened assessment of the client's presenting concerns and of therapeutic treatment.

To properly assess the impact of these images on client's self-view, therapists must actively engage and collaborate with their clients, because clients may not be aware of, or draw connections among, their behavior, belief systems, self-image, and these mythical images. Nevertheless, each therapeutic relationship should be approached with the awareness that, despite commonalities, the experiences of each Woman of Color are unique, and they are affected by such factors as socioeconomic status, educational background, family history, racial identity, and experience with racism (for example, individual experiences, what region of the country they grew up in) (Greene, 1994). Exploring the client's cultural reality by specifically asking about her unique experiences as a Woman of Color both facilitates the client's self-disclosure (C. E. Thompson, Worthington, & Atkinson, 1994) and shows respect for the client's unique background. Direct discussion with Black female clients about these socially constructed images of the SBW and the Jezebel and how these images may relate to their concerns, problems, depression, stressors, and therapeutic goals can lead to more meaningful and comprehensive assessments and interventions.

Finally, therapists can assist clients in reducing role strain in several ways. First, care must be taken to avoid perpetuating and reinforcing the Mammy image and the SBW who is always willing and able to selflessly meet the needs of others. Therapy should be a place where Women of Color clients can safely step out of this role by showing their true selves; their feelings, from joy to anger to sorrow; and their genuineness, vulnerability, and fear. Also, therapists can apply an interpersonal approach to reducing role strain, such as letting the Woman of Color know that she does not have to make concessions for her husband or child in therapy. Rather, she can focus on her own feelings, needs, and desires. This often allows her to begin self-focused healing.

The cultural expectation is often that Black women will serve as caretakers for siblings, parents, and other community members in times of distress. Rather than quickly labeling a client as "codependent" when she opts to assume this caretaking role, culturally sensitive therapists are aware of the roles Black women play and the expectations placed on them by their extended family and community. Therapy can be a place to discuss ways of remaining connected without becoming continual caretakers or enmeshed in unhealthy family dynamics. The opportunity to vent feelings of anger, frustration, or guilt associated with becoming more autonomous or surpassing the achievements of other family members and peers can also be very healing.

RECOMMENDATIONS

The appropriate use of Black feminist therapies with Women of Color requires literacy and competence on the part of therapists, academics, and researchers. The following recommendations are suggested for comrades and allies interested in using the Black feminist perspective in education and practice.

- Social work feminists and allies must have the courage to discuss and document their work on Black feminisms in the practice literature and in public forums, such as at conferences and other meetings on mental and social health. Therapists in the academy should participate in continuing education programs that seek to enhance their practice skills and competency in the Black feminist perspective.
- Therapists must acknowledge their own value system and its potential impact on Women of Color in practice. Specifically, therapists must be tuned in to diversity and the ways in which their own values shape the therapeutic process.
- Therapists must possess a willingness to validate the perceptions of racism, discrimination, and bias that Women of Color have experienced

in mental health and social service agencies, providing a space in which Women of Color can re-story their identified problems without feeling invalidated or dismissed.

CONCLUSION

As underscored in this chapter, it is clear that little inquiry exists on feminist therapy and Women of Color in therapy. Just as feminism has been compelled to develop a more inclusive discourse that acknowledges the full array of diversity among women and the impacts of oppression on women, mental health therapy will similarly need to evolve. A Black feminist perspective challenges the prevailing notion in therapy that gender is the only salient category of oppression and insists that the experiences of White women cannot be generalized to the development of therapeutic treatment strategies for Black women. The challenge in the 21st century is to put Black feminist theory into action in mental health practice.

A Black feminist perspective reflects an integrated analysis of race, gender, sexuality, and class in therapy and offers possibilities for working with Women of Color in a holistic framework. It offers practitioners a useful method of providing services from a strengths-based perspective, in contrast to traditional models of the prognostic course and treatment of trauma, stress, and coping among Women of Color. An important goal of practitioners is to attend to both individual and societal stressors, especially those influenced and exacerbated by experiences of oppression, in an effort to promote positive mental health outcomes among Women of Color. In addition, therapists should develop broad knowledge of community resources and encourage Women of Color to use these resources, as well as available spiritual, occupational, and family support systems.

These goals and opportunities provide a practical perspective for assisting Women of Color in healing the psychological and social damages of racism, sexism, and other forms of oppression that often obstruct self-actualizing behaviors. When progress is made, feminist therapeutic interventions may become more useful in assisting Black women to heal and recover. Black feminist therapy has the possibility of representing a beacon in therapeutic practice and serving as a political movement in combating the complex and simultaneous oppressions and psychosocial stressors faced by Women of Color. Such practice methods will not only help Women of Color reconstruct negative societal self-images formed by patriarchal therapeutic ideologies but also assist them in consciousness-raising regarding their socially constructed identities and rejecting socially induced shame and degradation.

The incorporation of Black feminist therapeutic perspectives that raise consciousness, foster resilience, and empower Women of Color will serve to decrease psychosocial stressors and promote positive coping strategies

(Boyd-Franklin, 2006; Greene, 1997; L. V. Jones & Ford, 2008; Vaz, 2005). Moreover, this mental health perspective will assist in cultivating modes of empowerment that Women of Color may use in the development of positive mental health outcomes. These modes of empowerment can include realization of one's potential, positive coping strategies, better quality of life, and positive influence on lifestyle and behavior (Greene, 1997; Jones & Ford, 2008; Taylor, 1998; Thomas & González-Prendes, 2009). Integral to the success of Black feminisms in therapeutic practice is the field's full-fledged commitment to creating positive mental health outcomes through its development of treatment protocols, delivery of services, and reaffirmation of its values. This commitment can promote equity and social justice for Women of Color and provide an invaluable framework for mental health practice and research for all oppressed groups.

CHAPTER QUESTIONS

1. How might you use Toni Cade Bambara's quote "Are you sure, sweetheart, that you want to be well? . . . Just so's you're sure, sweetheart, and ready to be healed, cause wholeness is no trifling matter. A lot of weight when you're well" in therapy with Women of Color?

2. What additional themes might come up in therapy with Women of Color? List the possible themes and discuss why.

3. Discuss your understanding of the Strong Black Women construct and provide examples relevant to your work/internship or clinical experience.

4. What additional therapy or counseling recommendations might you suggest when providing therapy to Women of Color?

CHAPTER 6

Case Illustrations

Black feminist therapy grows out of an ideological and philosophical stance: Black feminist praxis. The components of Black feminist therapy are the basic principles of this philosophy and ideology that are used in therapeutic processes and interventions. Hence, one of the most effective ways (other than through practice experience) to become proficient in Black feminist therapeutic praxis is to learn through the experience of Black feminist therapists. Black feminist therapy asks practitioners to be self-reflective, engage in knowledge building, and view women from their unique standpoint. What follows are case illustrations based on my clinical experience, using individual, group, and family modalities that highlight the basic components of Black feminist therapy as outlined in chapter 2. These case illustrations can be used to facilitate class discussion, role-plays, or other small-group exercises. In discussing the case illustrations or scenarios, the following questions can be used to structure dialogue:

- Briefly discuss the following gender–race factors in this Woman of Color's life and how they might be affecting the client's current life situations and psychosocial challenges:
  - How does U.S. culture define this person's role as a Woman of Color? What are the familial role expectations?
  - How do these gender–race role expectations influence this Woman of Color's relationships in the workplace, educational settings, social service institutions, and so forth?

- Reflect on the cultural values, worldviews, and assumptions you currently hold in relation to this Woman of Color and her presenting problem or problems. Discuss how your own multiple status affiliations—oppressed and privileged (for example, by gender, race, sexual orientation)—influence your assessment of this client's presenting concerns. What do you need to challenge yourself on or examine further to provide culturally competent services to this client?
- How might you use a Black feminist therapist perspective with this Women of Color?
  - Considering Black feminist philosophy and ideology, how might you reframe what's going on with this client?
  - What specific components of Black feminist therapy are critical for this case?
  - What types of mezzo- or macro-level interventions would benefit this client?
- What strengths of the client would you draw on when working with her? In what areas does the client need further empowerment?

Client: Mariela

Age: 22

Cultural, Ethnic, or Racial Group: Dominican American, Latina

Occupation: part-time sales manager

Presenting Problems: homelessness, history of alcohol and drug abuse, symptoms of depression, feelings of isolation

Phase of the Helping Process: engagement

Black Feminist Therapy Principles Used: consciousness-raising, empowerment

Mariela, a 16-year-old woman of Latin descent, left home where she had a strained relationship with her father and married Ricky Sr., age 22, whom she had been dating for six months. By age 18, Mariela had two children. During her third pregnancy, her husband became physically violent and psychologically abusive. Mariela decided that she "could not take it anymore, for me, for my kids." She put things in motion to move out. Because of her strained relationship with her father, she was forced to move into a family-based shelter program. Although the shelter program ensured her and her children's safety, Mariela had to relocate far away from her support system of friends and relatives. Mariela reported to her resident adviser that she felt alienated and isolated from other residents, and she stated, "My kids don't have any friends and I don't know anyone around here, and no one even speaks Spanish."

In search of companionship at the shelter, Mariela began looking for friends on the streets, where she began to experiment with drugs and drink alcohol. Over the course of several weeks, Mariela showed signs and behaviors of being distraught. Her resident adviser, Nelia, noticed that Mariela was very short-tempered with her children. In fact, she had yelled at her son Ricky Jr., "Stupid, you're just like your daddy, no good." One evening after the children's bedtime, Nelia decided to stop by Mariela's residence to check in with her. Nelia asked, "Are you okay?" and Mariela said, "Why do you say that? I will always be okay." As Nelia and Mariela sat together in silence, Mariela began to sob. "I feel like I'm going crazy," Mariela said. She asked Nelia if she knew someone who would "understand me, even look like me, someone I can talk to." By the next morning, Nelia had set up an urgent appointment with a local mental health clinic and asked that Mariela be matched with a Latina and or, if that was not possible, with any other Woman of Color therapist who spoke Spanish, in hopes of connecting her with a therapist who shared some of her cultural values.

Mariela was matched with Dr. Christina Simon, a Spanish-speaking, Dominican social worker. During the initial session, Mariela appeared to be withdrawn. Ten minutes into the session, Mariela noticed a beautiful print above Christina's desk and asked, pointing to it, "Dr. Simon, who is that picture of?" In an effort to make Mariela feel comfortable, Christina said, "Please call me Christina." Glancing at the print, she said, "Mariela, that is Queen Yuiza Loiza of the Taino people of Puerto Rico. She gave her life to protect her people. She took great risks beyond what was common. She was a hero and was greatly admired by her tribal people and continues to be, even today. Are you familiar with her?"

"Yeah, kinda," Mariela responded. "I remember my grandmother having a picture of her on the wall when I was little girl."

"What a powerful picture of strength to see as you were growing up," Christina said. She briefly shared the legend of Yuiza Loiza, the last Taino queen. Mariela listened attentively. After a short pause, Mariela said, "I just haven't had the strength to get there lately." With strong emotion and conviction, Mariela further revealed, "You know, it's so hard being a Latina. Society doesn't always respect you, and your family pressures you to succeed. And forget love and support from your husband. That's why I have become so angry, and it all soon led me down the path of drugs and alcohol. . . . I thought it would take the pain away, but, no, I have become explosive. . . . But my kids [as she pulled out a photo], I know they love me, and I love them, that's why I have to get my shit together."

Christina smiled and said, "There is something about you ... you seem to have the soul of a warrior, just like your Puerto Rican ancestor, Queen Yuiza Loiza. I think that we can do some great work together. What do you think?" A teardrop landed on Mariela's cheek as she nodded in agreement. "So, can we start by you sharing a bit more about what brought you here today? Where shall we start?"

Over the next three sessions, Christina used Black feminist principles of consciousness-raising and knowledge building to explore Mariela's struggles in a sociopolitical context. They discussed how racism and sexism affect Mariela and how understanding social context would help her build resilience. Christina was able to engage with Mariela by drawing on cultural traditions and beliefs, such as collective responsibility, that resonated with Mariela's life experiences and emphasized the strengths inherent in her cultural identity. In a similar vein, Christina worked to teach Mariela about Latino role models who had successfully negotiated difficult challenges in their lives and communities to provide her with a sense of hope and a vision for change. Through these strategies, Mariela received acknowledgment and validation of both her current and the historical (societal, cultural, and family) realities of Latina women's (and men's) devalued status in U.S. society and how they play out in her interpersonal relationships and in her current state of homelessness. In terms of assessment, Christina gained a greater understanding of Mariela's feelings of loss, disappointment, and shame surrounding her family. Mariela began to describe how her feelings of isolation led her to the dead-end street of drug experimentation. These themes resonate with concepts in the feminist therapy literature, pointing to the importance of a supportive, cohesive social context in promoting resilience. Mariela described how the lack of this supportive social context resulted in feelings of isolation, anger, hopelessness, and negative outcomes, including her need to leave her husband and her subsequent homelessness.

Christina began to create the conditions for resilience by establishing a sense of racial, cultural, and gender pride in talking about other women—in particular—Black and Brown Latina women—who have been able to overcome and survive difficulties such as abuse (physical and emotional), loss, and drug and alcohol addiction. She shared examples and asked Mariela to do the same. Mariela then recalled an aunt who overcame huge hurdles in her life: "My favorite aunt Melba used to be addicted to crack. She's been clean for 12 years. Evelyn Lozada and Ana Ortiz were able to re-establish themselves after being in physically and emotionally abusive relationships, and, of course, Whitney Houston. I don't know how it happened to her, but she fought the drug addiction battle, as well as the abuse. It was so sad when she died. And then her poor daughter died from an overdose too."

Christina further intervened by exploring the societal construction of Women of Color as caretakers and "superwomen" and how Women of Color had accepted these roles mainly as a result of the need to survive. She explained that, at one time, the superwoman role may have helped women and their families and communities to survive but that today this role has become a habit. "These myths date back to the days of slavery, when we had to ignore our emotional needs to survive." She further discussed how belief in the myth that Women of Color are invincible and can endure any adversity without breaking down is psychologically damaging. After giving this some thought, Mariela said, "I feel like I live that myth.... I only know how to take care of others these days and not myself." Christina then explained, "To reduce our psychological stressors, we must take a deep look into our reality and explore what we can and cannot control and what leads us to believe that we are always in control of our family's and friends' lives as well as our own. We just can't take on everybody and everything. We can only take on what we control in our own lives. And sometimes even that is hard."

In this dialogue, Christina used the Black feminist therapy method of consciousness-raising to demonstrate cultural competence and an understanding of the social and historical contexts that have influenced Mariela's behavior. This created the foundation for a therapeutic relationship in which Mariela could explore and apply coping strategies. This supportive relationship, combined with new coping strategies (for example, self-acceptance, dealing effectively with mistakes, positivity, development of a social network), was aimed at helping Mariela build resilience. Christina and Mariela continued to discuss past coping strategies that had been useful in times of distress, such as talking to someone, exercise, and meditation. Christina also offered tangible tools for addressing such issues as stress and internalized oppression.

As demonstrated in this case, counseling interventions informed by Black feminist principles provide therapists with tools that help them to understand and respond to the complexity of the experience of oppression faced across both the micro- and the macro-system levels. Mariela's hesitation to seek treatment and her statement that she will always be okay were rooted in the internalized tradition that says that Women of Color must be strong in the face of adversity.

Client: Nathalie

Age: 54

Cultural, Ethnic, or Racial Group: Guyanese

Occupation: design manager

Presenting Problems: anxiety, depression, and low self-esteem

Phase of the Helping Process: engagement and assessment

Black Feminist Principles Used: consciousness-raising, empowerment, race–gender role analysis

Nathalie is a 54-year-old married woman of Guyanese descent, with no children. She works for a local marketing firm as a design specialist and began to feel overwhelmed and frustrated with colleagues about her workload. Nathalie called her insurance company and requested a therapist of color. At the time of intake with the therapist, she reported a lack of self-esteem and symptoms of anxiety and depression.

In her first session, Nathalie said that although she knows that her husband, Chris, loves her, "He just doesn't always get me." She described her continual self-doubt, lack of self-esteem, and feelings of anxiety and depression as "feelings that keep me from interacting with my colleagues, and anyone else outside of my immediate family. I'm so embarrassed and afraid. My husband thinks I'm strange because I shy away from meeting new people. The White guys at my job don't even say hi or look my way; they think I'm stupid. But I'm smart. I have a master's degree in business marketing and accounting, and many of them don't. My parents make me feel this way too. Even though the other two Black women in my firm invite me out to lunch often, I just can't find the energy to say yes."

On the basis of the specific issues raised in the assessment process, the therapist engaged Nathalie in a race–gender role analysis and a power analysis to assist her in identifying issues that create and exacerbate her low self-confidence, anxiety, and depression (for example, social withdrawal, difficulty sleeping and eating, lack of motivation, expecting little out of life, and worrying about whether she has treated others badly).

Over sessions 2 and 3, Nathalie became comfortable, and she began discussing some of her self-identified problems. Nathalie reported that she experienced anxiousness, sweaty palms, heart pounding, and stuttering when asked to provide reports in meetings. In an attempt to avoid these symptoms, she kept quiet during meetings and made excuses or pretended to feel sick when she was scheduled to deliver a presentation. Accordingly, she regularly felt ashamed and embarrassed because her White male colleagues would often put her on the spot. She reported often becoming red in the face and tongue-tied because she worried about whether she had answered the question well enough. She also worried about how she was perceived afterward. In contrast, she described herself as smart, hardworking, and one who "has made many contributions to the company." Yet she wondered why she had low self-esteem and self-confidence despite her significant abilities and accomplishments.

During the engagement and assessment processes, Nathalie brought up many issues that were sensitive and important to her. She was raised in a middle-class, religious family. She is the firstborn and has two younger brothers. She said that her parents favored her two brothers, Christopher and Edmund, and always told her to "follow their good examples for almost everything I did ... their study skills, basketball, easygoing ways with friends and adults, how well they expressed their ideas, their lively personalities, everything!" She also shared that she felt that her parents liked her husband more than they liked her. Needless to say, she resented all of this.

Although she had earned her master's degree, worked at a good-paying job in a respectable profession, was an excellent cook, and had developed plenty of skills that proved her intelligence and excellence, her parents still gave her brothers and husband more attention and often raved at family gatherings about how successful they were (Christopher is a computer technician, and Edmond is a lawyer). There was never a word spoken about her job or achievements. In addition, she recalled situations from her early childhood when she was "imitating others" and "acting as she thought her brothers would" to gain her parents' and teachers' acceptance and recognition. She also related several sarcastic remarks from her parents and brothers about her physical appearance (for example, "You're getting fat," "What are you doing with your hair?") and job choice (for example, "You're not going to make any money in marketing"). She shared that her only defense was to "withdraw from socializing with them or anyone when she experienced injustice and rejection."

As her therapy sessions continued, she realized that withdrawal had become her way of coping. She and her therapist discussed withdrawal as a means to get attention and the ways in which her whole life revolved around trying to achieve recognition, acceptance, and value from her parents. In an attempt to get her parents' attention, she made it her duty to become "a very good daughter, an excellent cook and housewife, plus a great professional." None of this gave her inner peace or satisfaction. In the engagement and assessment process, the therapist explained the importance of conducting a gender–race analysis along with a Black feminist analysis.

Therapy at this point was directed toward Nathalie's awareness of the gender–race roles that she had learned in her socialization process. Nathalie and her therapist tackled this concern, and Nathalie became aware of the assumed, subjectively structured female and male rights; in particular, Black female rights and Black women's position in society. Time was also spent talking about religion and the role of the church in Black families. These beliefs can frequently affect Black women's self-esteem. Nathalie's personal attitudes, such as "I am not worthy and I am not good because I am a Black and female," had a negative impact on her self-esteem and self-worth. Nathalie came to realize that her efforts and fights for others, her focus on others' rights, and her sensitivity to others came from a place of feeling devalued herself. In her deep desire to have her own worth valued by her parents, she was "acting and imitating" in ways that she thought would elicit their acknowledgment and recognition.

Natalie also realized that, because of her powerless position as a Black woman, she reacted to injustice and rejection by "being stoic and rigid with colleagues." Her inner wish was to "feel loved and accepted" and to be recognized as a magnificent, beloved, and valuable individual "beyond my race and gender." She wondered, "Why not? I'm a good and valuable Black woman." When she became aware of this, Nathalie's symptoms of extreme self-consciousness, self-doubt, and heart palpitations receded. She felt more confident and happier. She did not worry as much about whether people liked her because she was more confident in everything she said and did.

Over the next several sessions, Nathalie and her therapist focused on identifying internalized gender- and race-related messages and discussed alternative ways of knowing and being. As a result of her parents' preference for "their boys," her internalized message was "I can't do anything good enough because I am a stupid girl, not as good as my brothers. I'm useless to my parents and at work." Her therapist attempted to restructure these beliefs with self-affirming messages about her strengths, skills, and talents. She was able to communicate with her therapist about her negative feelings and dissatisfaction with males in general, especially her brothers and those at work who often dismissed her ideas in meetings. She further discussed with her therapist ways in which her work environment could become a place to start over and develop relationships with other Women of Color who desired to engage with her.

Through consciousness-raising regarding her family dynamics and self-perceptions of the role she plays in the family, Nathalie also began valuing her inner self when she was with her family and, more broadly, in social situations. This led her to the realization of male bias and the myth of proper positioning in relation to self, family, and society. She became aware of her rage toward and disappointment with her parents. She managed to forgive them by recognizing that "they did the best they could do in raising me, but now that I am aware of these underlying biases, I won't repeat their mistakes." Nathalie's sessions closed with her expressing, "I feel powerful and more confident now; I am able to link my behavior to my inner feelings, and I am able to replace these behaviors with my real needs and communicate them."

This case study illustrates the impact of Black feminist therapeutic tactics of conducting a race–gender role analysis and consciousness-raising about how familial and societal perceptions and actions via psychological darts can have a negative impact on Women of Color's social development and self-esteem. The application of Black feminist therapy goals and principles resulted in positive therapeutic outcomes in this case. The case also demonstrates and affirms the value of Black feminist theory and practice.

Client: Lola

Age: 32

Cultural, Ethnic, or Racial Identity: African American

Occupation: unemployed, former vice president at a technology firm

Presenting Problem: depression

Phase of the Helping Process: working phase

Black Feminist Principles Used: consciousness-raising, empowerment, race–gender role analysis

Lola is a 32-year-old African American woman; a mother of two, ages seven and 12; and separated from her spouse. She recently lost her job as a vice president of development at a technology firm. At intake she stated, "I committed myself to my job, I gave them three miserable years of my life, and they just told me in a five-minute meeting that they were moving in a different direction." She reported poor sleeping and eating patterns, tearfulness, decreased energy, and difficulty concentrating over the past few months.

Lola chose a Black women's therapy group for her treatment. In her first two sessions, Lola rarely participated in group conversations without prompting and did not offer feedback to the other participants. The third session of the group focused on stress and coping in the lives of African American women. During this session, the group leader provided a definition of psychological stress. The group leader then asked the members to identify their various emotional and physical reactions to stress. Members voiced several reactions, such as "I lose my patience," "I can't breathe," "I feel overwhelmed," "I feel exhausted," "I get irritable," "I eat too much," and "I feel like I'm having a nervous breakdown." The group leader asked members to identify possible stressors related to them as Black women. Lola suddenly spoke up: "Since our first meeting y'all been whining about how your boss treats you, you're always letting this shit get in your way. You'll need to bulldoze down your issues and the people in your way. You have no control over these negative things that happen."

Group members glared at Lola with disappointment and annoyance. A participant responded, "If you were perfect, you wouldn't be here." The group immediately responded in agreement. This brash statement seemed to encourage Lola to further open up: "Have you ever been in love with a man who didn't love you, so you looked for love in your work? Have you ever been stripped of your hard work and dedication and have not one soul to confide in? When you experience these things, come see me."

Despite their annoyance with her, group members listened attentively as Lola told her story, one filled with rejection and pain. Lola's narrative was rooted in the unfortunate internalized tradition that says that African American women must be strong in the face of adversity and accept life's ups and downs as products of their unalterable destiny.

The group leader provided support for Lola's story, noting that it illustrated how societal attitudes and biases can negatively influence a person's self-esteem and limit opportunities, resulting in a sense of powerlessness, suffering, sadness, anger, and anxiety. The group leader said, "An important part of our work here is identifying our strengths and the positive ways in which we can cope with daily life adversities. One way is through support of one another, so we'll start that here. Let's back up and identify the external stressors that we are reacting to, and that in turn cause us pain."

She also explained that as harmful beliefs and judgments are identified and feelings of anger and disappointment are worked through, women can feel a greater self-confidence, acceptance, and satisfaction in life and in relationships. The group leader concluded by encouraging group members to support each other as they worked through their issues in the group: "We must work toward liberating ourselves from deep sadness, using this group as a forum to become connected with our feelings and to tell our stories. If you can tell your story, we can help each of you."

By the end of the session, the group members began to understand, identify with, and support Lola. Lola became less defensive and more open to receiving feedback from the group for the remainder of the support group program. The support offered by the group members gave Lola and the other women tangible tools to address difficulties with stress, relationships, work, and money and help each other see how their internalized oppression held them back.

Client: Angel

Age: 38

Cultural, Ethnic, or Racial Group: African American

Occupation: housewife

Presenting Problems: interpersonal violence, involvement of Child Protective Services (CPS)

Phase of the Helping Process: investigation

Black Feminist Therapy Principles Used: sensitivity in assessment, race–power gender analysis

Angel is a 38-year-old African American mother of one, and she has been married to her spouse, Chris, for nine years. A CPS case was recently opened on the family after Chris was arrested after an incident of domestic violence: Chris pushed Angel down the cellar stairs at their home during an argument about his drinking. The police were called by the couple's seven-year-old daughter, Amaya, who witnessed the incident. Jackie, a woman of African descent and veteran CPS worker, was assigned to work with the family.

At the initial home visit, Angel shared with Jackie that as young children, she and her brother Ricky were removed from her mother's custody and placed in nonrelative foster care. Angel reported that her mother struggled with major depression, anxiety, and alcoholism, which she never sought help for because "you don't discuss your business outside the family." Angel further shared, "When I was a child [seven to nine years old], the police and ambulance would come to my house often; many times they would take my mother to the hospital for trying to hurt herself. My father and grandmother would expect me to take care of my little brother [three years old]; I was only a kid myself."

In frustration, Angel repeated the resonating words of the caseworker who removed her and her brother from their home: "They told my parents that they didn't have appropriate caretakers for their children." She went on to explain that despite numerous family members expressing a desire to open their homes to Angel and Ricky, they were placed into foster care. Neither she nor her brother were ever reunified with their mother. After conveying her family's history, Angel stated, "This can't be happening again. I don't even know why CPS is here. I already filed criminal charges against Chris, got a restraining order, and scheduled an appointment for Amaya to meet with the school counselor." Angel verbalized that she is terrified that CPS is going to tear her family apart: "You say you're here because you want to make sure Amaya's safe, but what you're really gonna do is take her away from me the first chance you get! I've seen this too many times, Black women in this community lose their children."

Using the Black feminist casework principle of demonstrating sensitivity in the investigation process, Jackie intervened by saying, "I hear you. I hear that you're afraid. I want you to know that I am not only here to make sure Amaya is safe, but I am also here to provide support for you. Can we work together to best understand what you both need to be safe?"

By the end of the meeting, Angel acknowledged that she needed support and agreed to work with Jackie. Reframing plays a vital role in investigation and service planning in child welfare cases.

Jackie was keenly aware of the power dynamics and inequality in the relationship between herself and Angel and was mindful as she proceeded with a race–gender role analysis. Jackie was a county CPS worker with the authority to take a child into care; Angel was a Black woman, a survivor of domestic violence, mother, and foster care alumna who was terrified of losing her daughter to the state. Considering power dynamics in the worker–parent relationship, Jackie knew that it was important to understand mothers from a place of strength, resilience, and empowerment and to understand the system from a place of historical inequality.

During the initial meeting, it became evident to Jackie that Angel had taken concrete steps to protect her daughter but that she was also vulnerable given her recent trauma, survivorship, and status as a Black woman. Acknowledging Angel's multiple oppressions as a caregiver in a demanding context required empathy. Jackie knew that responding with genuineness and an openness to change would allow Angel to share her concerns about services and treatment honestly, providing Jackie with the opportunity to remove barriers and resolve fears.

Over the next 30 days, Jackie met with Angel and Amaya on three additional occasions. During these visits, Jackie and Angel spent time negotiating their relationship and addressing issues of power, gender, and race. As a result of Angel's childhood experience with CPS and the belief that all CPS workers are "baby snatchers," she had developed a fear of CPS that informed how she interacted with CPS workers. Jackie began the assessment interview by initiating a race–gender role analysis with Angel, stating "I want to get a better idea of how you have been affected by family and societal demands." This analysis achieved two goals: First, Jackie learned more in-depth, specific information about Angel's worldview as a Woman of Color. Second, beginning with a race–gender role analysis allowed Angel to start to separate her personal goals, dreams, and expectations for herself from familial and societal goals and expectations. Jackie continued to use a race–gender analysis to better understand Angel's unique needs as a survivor of foster care and of domestic violence. The race–gender role analysis allowed Angel to recognize how gender role expectations and myths of Black women—her own and others'—affected her thoughts, actions, and feelings.

During their second and third meetings, Jackie worked with Angel to identify the race–gender role messages she had internalized as a child and young adult. Jackie helped Angel to examine her internalized belief that as a Black woman and mother, she must be a superwoman and take care of everyone in her family without asking for help or support in return. In addition, they discussed how Angel might hold on to helpful and needed cultural messages and values and learn to discard those that have a negative impact on her life; for example, the need to be strong for her husband even if he is abusive. With Angel's permission, Jackie verified from collateral providers that Angel had filed criminal charges, obtained a restraining order, and scheduled an intake appointment for Amaya at the community mental health clinic. At the end of their third meeting, Angel smiled with joy as Jackie stated, "No further intervention is warranted at this time because there are no safety or danger concerns."

Although Jackie's work with Angel was brief and limited to the completion of the initial assessment, attempts were made to restructure these beliefs with self-affirming messages about Angel's strengths, skills, and abilities. Through Jackie and Angel's work conducting a race–gender role analysis of how dominant family, cultural, and societal norms affected her sense of self and self-esteem, Angel successfully navigated the secondary trauma of having a CPS case opened after an incident of domestic violence. This case illustrates the impact of using Black feminist therapeutic principles in the context of CPS casework as a tool for engaging with clients who have experienced interpersonal and historical trauma and helping to facilitate strengths-based practice.

CHAPTER 7

Claiming Your Connections: An Evidence-Based Psychosocial Competence Group Intervention Grounded in Black Feminism

Having encountered a number of Women of Color in therapy with issues of psychosocial adjustment, depressive symptomatology, and external stressors and being aware of their limited opportunities to engage in culturally relevant interventions, I developed the Claiming Your Connections (CYC) group intervention program.

CYC is designed to expand opportunities for Women of Color in mental health therapy to engage in culturally congruent therapeutic interventions. The culturally congruent nature of the intervention protocol is based on treatment techniques that both directly and indirectly address specific aspects of Women of Color's psychosocial experiences in the United States (Belgrave, Chase-Vaughn, Gray, Addison, & Cherry, 2000; Miranda et al., 2003). *Cultural congruence* refers to (a) the integration of cultural attitudes, beliefs, and values of Women of Color into the intervention and (b) the continuous promotion of skills, practices, and interactions throughout the group process to ensure that sessions are culturally responsive and competent.

The CYC group intervention homes in on the outcomes of decreasing external locus of control and increasing active coping from a culturally relevant perspective on the basis of the needs and experiences of Women of Color. In the spirit of mutual aid, the outcomes of psychosocial competence are achieved in the CYC group intervention program by, first, providing members with an opportunity for self-exploration; second, providing members with the opportunity to acknowledge and validate both their current and their historical realities of unrecognized or devalued relationships, denigration of success, and undue destructive criticism of normative difficulties from the perspective of Women of Color's experiences; third, assisting members to identify unhealthy coping patterns; and fourth, teaching problem-solving and coping skills that promote an active stance of personal control and responsibility over their life goals and outcomes. A model is presented in this chapter.

This innovative group treatment model differs from traditional mental health approaches in that it provides a philosophical and treatment approach that incorporates the values and worldviews of racially and ethnically diverse populations (L. V. Jones, Ahn, & Chan, 2014; S. J. Jones, 2003) and may be specifically relevant for Women of Color. In addition to placing psychosocial competence at the forefront of the CYC model, this model explores the etiology of mental health difficulties using a Black feminist perspective. Using this perspective allows for a better understanding of the intersection and influence of race, gender, and class in the lives of Women of Color experiencing mental health disorders. Black feminism offers a model for practice that addresses the simultaneity of oppressions experienced by Women of Color, and it provides a framework for understanding modes of empowerment cultivated by Women of Color for psychological survival (L. C. Jackson & Greene, 2000). Given its focus on positive coping strategies and empowerment, psychosocial competence has tremendous resonance with the Black feminist perspective. Moreover, this model introduces literature authored by Women of Color as a tool to enhance ethnically and culturally specific group treatment. Because of the intervention's applicability across populations (for example, prevention, child welfare, juvenile justice, substance abuse treatment, and health care), the expectation is that the literature will be of interest to a diverse audience without losing its critical mass and social–psychological focus.

PSYCHOSOCIAL COMPETENCE: IMPLICATIONS FOR WOMEN OF COLOR

The emergent psychosocial competence model in mental health represents an innovative paradigm with potential relevance and applicability to preventing stress-related disorders among Women of Color. Psychosocial competence is consistent with newer conceptualizations of social work practice in which well-being is no longer equated with the absence of pathology but rather is seen as reflecting the presence of skills, knowledge, and qualities that enable a person to interact and function effectively within their ecological environment (Austin, 2000; Maluccio, Washitz, & Libassi, 1999; Tyler, Brome, & Williams, 1991).

In social work, as in other fields, *psychosocial competence* is defined as an individual's ability to function effectively at the personal, interpersonal, social, and task levels (L. V. Jones et al., 2014; Maluccio et al., 1999). Psychosocial competence is derived from the ecological paradigm for viewing human functioning, which draws from such fields as psychodynamic psychology; cognitive anthropology; and family systems, organizational, and learning and developmental theories (Maluccio et al., 1999). Although an ecological framework provides a way of conceptualizing and understanding human beings and their functioning in the context of their environment, research about competence development offers specific guidelines for professional practice and service delivery. Psychosocial competence is not a complete departure from earlier conceptualizations of understanding human behavior that have been embraced by practitioners and scholars. The psychosocial competence perspective is a modification of traditional theories that assume human functioning to be universal and predictable. Going beyond traditional theories, psychosocial competence addresses the way individuals perceive and interpret experience, providing a lens through which professionals can view their client's frames of reference to avoid or minimize cultural bias and to foster client growth.

Tyler (1978) proposed the psychosocial competence configuration as a way of examining different patterns of human functioning that characterize an individual's self-attitudes, worldviews, and behavioral attributes. Psychosocial competence promotes effective functioning in human beings by focusing on their unique coping and adaptive patterns: actual or potential strengths, natural helping networks, life experiences, and environmental resources as major instruments of intervention (Tyler, 1978). Tyler has hypothesized that in benign and predictable environments, more psychosocially competent people will be relatively self-efficacious, moderately trusting, and actively planful in their approaches to negotiating life events. In destructive, oppressive, or unpredictable environments, more psychosocially competent individuals will modify their self-worldviews and their approaches to events accordingly. In this configuration, individuals create for themselves a sense of self, a consciousness of their relationship to the world, and a way of negotiating life events in light of those perspectives (Tyler et al., 1991). Studies have demonstrated that different racial and ethnic groups have their own ways of building and integrating the components of psychosocial competence (Jarama, Belgrave, & Zea, 1996; L. V. Jones et al., 2014; Tyler & Sinha, 1988; Zea, Reisen, Beil, & Caplan, 1997). This conceptualization provides a model of practice that accepts different ways of coping and adapting as valid in the therapeutic process (Tyler et al., 1991). It recognizes that race and gender carry with them historical legacies, survival value, and a particular way of life. Hence, such a practice perspective uses these self-world behavioral attributes to gain a better understanding of the intersection and influence of race and gender in the lives of Women of Color.

Although a paucity of intervention research exists in the area of psychosocial competence and Women of Color, the few existing studies have supported the presence of a shared constellation of personal attributes in individuals who successfully negotiate life with all its unexpected changes (D. Evans & Tyler, 1976; Jarama et al., 1996; L. V. Jones et al., 2014; Zea et al., 1997). These findings suggest that during times of stress and adversity, or when Women of Color are confronted with less predictable environmental situations, interventions aimed at enhancing their sense of psychosocial competence may promote a more optimal pattern of functioning and promote greater well-being. Thus, Women of Color are more likely to develop a personality and behavioral pattern that is characterized by strengths, capabilities, and resilience and is more adaptive to alternative circumstances. Psychosocial competence also emphasizes concepts of independence, self-management, meaningful connection to others, and reliance on natural community supports (Tyler, 2002). Each of these notions has tremendous resonance with the worldviews and culture of Women of Color, further suggesting that psychosocial competence is a paradigm worth examining in Women of Color at risk of severe and persistent mental health disorders.

UNIQUENESS OF THE CYC CURRICULUM OPERATING FROM A BLACK FEMINIST PERSPECTIVE

Black feminist theory offers a good opportunity to more clearly understand the intersection and influence of racism, sexism, and class oppression in the lives of Women of Color (Collins, 2000). The Black feminist perspective provides a more salient way to account for how the cumulative effects created by the multiple role conflicts experienced by Women of Color can result in emotional isolation and stress-related symptoms. Although both the Afrocentric and feminist perspectives in psychology were developed to challenge cultural ideologies that universalize traits of Black people and women, theorists have largely failed to integrate the diversity of these experiences into their theories for those whose experiences do not conform to these cultural models (Gardner & Enns, 2004). For instance, feminist models have traditionally mirrored characteristics of educated White women, yet these models use language that universalizes these characteristics to all women (L. C. Jackson & Greene, 2000). Similarly, Afrocentric theory does not distinguish the experience of Women of Color from that of the "generic" African American, that is, male (Asante, 1992; Nobles, 1991). Thus, the experiences of Women of Color are viewed using a perspective that may account for culture but does not incorporate Women of Color's different experiences of oppression. Many theorists and researchers have increased their efforts to transcend universalization and the limitations of Afrocentric and feminist psychology to be more inclusive of race and class in the development of the Black feminist (Braun-Williams, 1999).

Black feminism's emphasis on emotional wholeness, psychological strength, and resilience—and their centrality to Women of Color's historical struggles—has remained at the core of Black feminist theory. Rather than focusing on individual psychopathology, Black feminist theory posits that oppression such as racism, sexism, and classism is an important aspect of Women of Color's psychological distress. King (1988) asserted that the social construction of these oppressions constitutes three interdependent control systems that are interactive and produce unique, multiple-jeopardy situations for Women of Color. Following this logic, Women of Color's greater likelihood of having stress-related mental health disorders would be seen as an inevitable result of the many conflicts they face as they navigate multiple roles and identities on a daily basis. For instance, depression among Women of Color should be seen as an outgrowth of multiple conflicting socially defined roles and identities, and a true understanding of the nature of depression in this population is best gained from reshaping one's view from one of pathology to one of quiet sacrifice. Thus, intervention strategies based on Black feminist principles are more likely to be effective because they account for the complexity of Women of Color's life experiences. Interventions should therefore aim at assisting Women of Color to sort out the personal from the contextual by helping them recognize how internalization of socially constructed identities has contributed to their stress-related symptoms (C. B. Williams, 2005). Ultimately, interventions should be designed to assist Women of Color in recognizing and changing unhealthy elements of their lives.

GROUP WORK WITH WOMEN OF COLOR

Significant changes in psychosocial competency can be generated through an array of intervention modalities, including individual, family, or group treatment. Group treatment is particularly promising because it can integrate different treatment strategies to achieve social support, skill development, and role change (Toseland & Rivas, 2017). In particular, group work can establish a context in which participants learn new coping skills using didactic techniques, role modeling, and information sharing.

In homogeneous group settings in which Women of Color are significantly underrepresented, conscious and unconscious group dynamics of mainstreaming and devaluation of differences can undermine needed therapeutic work (Garvin, Gutierrez, & Galinsky, 2017). Being the only racial or ethnic minority, gay, or female group member can be isolating and may make it difficult to relate to others in the group. Minority members may question their own judgment. They may also feel inferior or pressured to agree with the majority. For these reasons, minority members may derive less benefit from the group (Fenster, 1996). However, heterogeneous groups may provide a natural and less stigmatizing context for help seeking than other forms of mental health treatment (Denton, 1990; Gutierrez, 1990; Hopps & Pinderhughes, 1999). It has been posited that group practice aimed at intervening with Women of Color may decrease isolation and increase support by fostering interaction, affiliation, and social involvement among group members (Boyd-Franklin, 1991; Denton, 1990; Hopps et al., 1995).

Women of Color have participated in a variety of formal and informal support groups for social, psychological, and economic reasons (Short & Williams, 2014). The acts of support, care taking, and educating one another through groups is a cultural phenomenon that has been used throughout history by Women of Color and their communities (for examples, see L. V. Jones & Warner, 2011). Support groups were used to affirm and acknowledge their non-nurturing, hostile social and psychological realities and to offer the opportunity to assist one another in coping with the consequent psychological distress. Hence, when working with Women of Color, it is important to integrate their worldviews and expectations: Appreciate the dynamics of Black culture and its influence on optimal mental health, recognize thematic cultural beliefs and values, and understand the impact of such beliefs and values on group work (Pack-Brown & Fleming, 2004).

Descriptions of group interventions and techniques related to race or culture, specifically as they pertain to Women of Color and enhancement of psychosocial competence, are few in the research and practice literatures. This omission may, in part, be due to the fact that group work research has been traditionally devoted to the development of universal conceptualizations that supposedly guide all group practice (see Yalom, 2005, for detailed discussion of group theory and dynamics). The oversight of race and culture as salient factors in the development of group theory has resulted in the omission of unique experiences and specific needs of Women of Color from group process and outcomes (Hopps & Pinderhughes, 1999). Although there is no "best" model of group work practice for Black clients, there is a recognition that Black people, like other ethnic or racial groups, are neither attitudinally nor behaviorally monolithic and therefore cannot be approached with a singular method of intervention. It has been posited that group work has the potential to serve as an effective intervention for the reduction of stress symptoms and the enhancement of psychosocial competence with Women of Color.

USE OF LITERARY WORKS IN GROUP WORK

Surviving and thriving despite life's stresses often requires new ways of thinking about and relating to the social environment. For Women of Color who experience low levels of emotional well-being, the CYC intervention builds on the strengths perspective that psychosocial competence is relevant to providing treatment services for depression that are culturally congruent. Evidence has suggested that mental health interventions that focus on the psychosocial competence of Women of Color would do well to incorporate culturally congruent methods that simultaneously empower participants while speaking to their needs as Women of Color. One such method may be engagement in literary dialogue written by and about Women of Color. Literary works that emphasize the collective struggles of Women of Color demystify the treatment process and provide a forum for working through issues in group settings that encourages cultural identity and Black well-being.

The use of literary works, or bibliotherapy, in mental health interventions constitutes a process of dynamic interaction between the reader and the literature (Maidman Joshua & DiMenna, 2000). Its use in group interventions is reported to be useful with people across age groups, in outpatient and inpatient settings, and with healthy people who want to share their interpretations of literature as a means of personal growth and development (L. V. Jones & Hodges, 2002). The use of literary works in mental health treatment is a process that addresses not only emotional problems but also less complicated issues facing people in their everyday lives. Recent research has provided support for its effectiveness (L. V. Jones, 2000; L. V. Jones & Hodges, 2002; L. V. Jones & Warner, 2011; Shechtman, 2000). L. V. Jones et al. (2014) found that the use of bibliotherapy had a positive impact on attitude change, assertiveness, and self-development and affected other forms of psychosocial gain. Riordan and Wilson (1989) reported change in inappropriate behaviors, improved self-esteem, and interpersonal growth and development. Bibliotherapy has also been found to be effective in increasing feelings of self-worth and self-efficacy among adults with depression (Cuijpers, 1998). Given these positive findings, literature clearly constitutes a useful treatment tool for enhancing group work.

In addition to providing an effective technique for intervening with the population of Women of Color, the use of literature in this group model reaches beyond traditional methods of treatment toward affirming and integrating the values and worldviews of People of Color. Consistent with psychosocial competence development, the use of literary works facilitates the group process by enabling self-identification with others, by prompting women to give and receive feedback, and by encouraging them to face personal challenges. Once members can identify and process themes in the readings that have played a negative or positive role in their own lives, they are able to raise these issues for discussion in relation to their own personal experiences. Overall, the use of literature in the group process allows members to see Women of Color in the readings survive by adjusting, readjusting, and adapting to an ever-changing reality.

LEADING CYC GROUPS

Group development is helpful in providing guidance to facilitators on group dynamics and the actual unfolding of the group process over time. Facilitators should not assume that all groups follow the same developmental pattern and reach optimal functioning at the same rate. Many structural and functional characteristics affect a group's development, such as whether a group is open-ended or closed-ended, heterogeneous or homogeneous, or time-limited (Toseland, Jones, & Gellis, 2004). Similarly, the support of the initiating agency or organization can also affect elements of group process and development. All of these characteristics can influence group member satisfaction and, ultimately, the level of success the group will have in attaining its goals. Although individual and environmental characteristics may strongly influence the development of the group, the focus here is on the regularity and consistencies of group development.

Five Phases of Group Work

Reviews of group development practice and research have supported the idea that group dynamics evolve over time (Toseland & Rivas, 2017). Although there are many widely used models of group development (namely, Bales, 1965; Garland, Jones, & Kolodny, 1976), the CYC model centers on Tuckman's (1965) sequential stage model of group development that is most frequently cited in the group literature. Tuckman provided a model of group development that fits well with the phases of group work in social work settings. He concluded that groups go through five predictable developmental stages over time: forming, storming, norming, performing, and adjourning. (For a more detailed list and description of group development models, see Toseland & Rivas, 2017.)

Forming. The central process during the forming stage of group development is focused on orientation to clarify common goals and values and to determine the group's structure, which increases group stability. Members become oriented to the group by attempting to identify behaviors acceptable to the leader and other group members (see, for example, Mann, Gibbard, & Hartman, 1967). Serious issues and feelings are avoided, and people focus on being busy with routines, such as team organization, task assignment, and scheduling. Leaders assist members to develop a sense of trust in the group and help develop the norms under which the group will operate. For example, during the initial stage, facilitators can help build trust and create a more relaxed group environment by emphasizing the importance of confidentiality about what is shared in the group.

Storming. During the storming phase, management of conflict often becomes the focus of attention (see, for example, Yalom, 2005). Conflicts frequently erupt over issues of power, authority, and competition within the group regarding task accomplishment (Harris & Sherblom, 2008). Most important, very little communication occurs because no one is listening, and some are still unwilling to talk openly. At this stage, group facilitators will need to enforce skills that assist the group to negotiate conflict. For example, facilitators will need to assist members in expressing their thoughts and feelings toward others in a respectful manner. This includes active listening without interrupting others to disagree. Facilitators can also ask members to use "I" statements in communicating their feelings and thoughts rather than speaking in the second person. Several theories suggest that if conflicts are adequately resolved during this stage, members' relationships with the leader and with each other become more trusting and cohesive (Tuckman & Jensen, 1977). Energy devoted to developing cohesive group functioning and comfortable norms and productive roles in earlier group meetings gives way to productive interaction during the norming phase of group work.

Norming. The norming stage is characterized by members' commitment to exploring the significant problems they bring to the sessions. At this point in a group's evolution, facilitators find that the degree of structuring and intervention is lower than during the forming stage. Moreover, this stage in the developmental sequence is devoted to the development of trust and more mature and open negotiation regarding roles, group structure, and division of labor. Having had their disagreements, group members now understand each other better and can appreciate the skills and experiences each brings to the group process. Individuals listen to each other, appreciate and support each other, and are prepared to change preconceived views and notions.

Performing. During the performing stage, members develop proficiency in achieving goals and become more flexible in their patterns of teamwork. Group identity, loyalty, and morale are all high, and everyone is equally task oriented and committed to carrying out assigned roles and responsibilities. Group facilitators can help members clarify their tasks and make assignments on the basis of members' talents and interests.

Adjourning. During the adjourning stage, groups finish their tasks, make decisions, and produce the results of their efforts. The adjourning stage is also vital for members because they have the opportunity to bring closure to remaining tasks, clarify the meaning of their experiences in the group, consolidate their gains, and decide what newly acquired skills and behaviors they want to transfer into their everyday lives. For many group members and leaders, endings are difficult because they realize that their time in group is limited. This stage often triggers memories of other losses that members have experienced. Thus, termination of the group often entails a grieving process. It is important that leaders identify and explore feelings that permeate the culture.

Engaging Group Diversity

Practitioners must raise their level of awareness about the issues facing Women of Color in the real world and how these dynamics unfold in the group process. Specifically, practitioners must be aware of how the intersections of race, gender, and class influence Women of Color's perceptions of mental health and how to incorporate this awareness into the group work process.

Valuing Individual Members. The values, preferences, and interpersonal styles of individual members that come from their ethnic, cultural, and racial heritage; previous life experiences; and genetic disposition have to be blended together before a group culture develops. As members meet, they explore their value systems and interpersonal styles, searching for a common ground on which to relate to each other. Valuing members from diverse backgrounds involves leaders facilitating an exploration of members' ethnic and racial heritages and experiences, their attitudes about themselves, and how these attitudes and feelings affect their functioning. It also involves leaders actively generating a set of group norms that are consonant with the cultural values and perspectives of all group members (Short & Williams, 2014). As a result of this process, a common set of assumptions, values, and preferred ways of doing business emerge, forming the group's culture.

Valuing Diversity. Multicultural differences are also salient interpersonal factors that have significance for the group culture. Traditionally, group processes have reflected the European and American values of individualism, independence, competitiveness, and achievement. These values are different from the values of humility and modesty that are dominant in other cultures. A potential consequence is the therapist's insensitivity to group members from other racial or ethnic backgrounds. This insensitivity has the potential to negatively affect group dynamic processes in the whole group.

Racially and ethnically diverse groups tend to have their own cultural attributes, values, and experiences as a result of their unique histories. Cultural experiences of group survival, social hierarchy, inclusiveness, and ethnic identification influence the way members interact with one another in the group. In a multicultural group, members' expectations and goals vary widely, and they significantly influence the dynamics of the group (Matsukawa, 2001). To be effective with all group members, the group leader should be sensitive to racial, ethnic, and socioeconomic differences; understand the effect of these differences on group dynamics; and translate this knowledge into culturally sensitive modes of program development and service delivery.

Group Culture. A distinct culture tends to emerge more quickly in groups that are homogeneous. When members share similar values and life experiences, their unique perspectives blend more quickly than in groups with diverse membership. For example, a caregiver support group made up of the spouses of frail veterans tends to form a distinct culture more quickly than a caregiver support group made up of both spouses and adult children who are caring for frail older people who have not all shared military service.

Conversely, heterogeneous groups offer opportunities to provide and receive diverse feedback to develop more knowledge and understanding of oneself and others and to develop the skills needed to relate to people of different backgrounds (Fenster, 1996; Merta, 1995). However, if facilitated inappropriately, heterogeneous multicultural groups run the risk of re-enacting oppressive dynamics of invalidation, disempowerment, lack of empathy, and mutuality. Therefore, it is important that group leaders be informed, attuned, and adept at processing the roles of race, culture, ethnicity, and power (Pinderhughes, Jackson, & Romney, 2017).

Avoiding Member Isolation. Once a culture has developed, members who endorse and share in the group culture feel at home, but those who do not feel isolated and alienated. For the isolated member, the group is not a very satisfying experience. Isolated members are more likely to leave the group because it does not meet their socioemotional needs. Feeling misunderstood and left out is demoralizing and depressing. More extreme feelings of alienation can lead to rebellious, acting-out behavior. For subgroups who are not part of the dominant culture, feelings of isolation are often equated with feelings of oppression. Subgroups who feel repressed are likely to rebel in various ways against the norms, roles, and status hierarchies that have been established in the group. By providing individual attention to isolated members, and by stimulating all members to consider values that transcend individual differences, leaders can foster the full participation and integration of all group members into the group.

CYC GROUP MODEL: FORMAT AND PROCESS

CYC involves a weekly counseling group to enhance psychosocial competency skills using a cognitive therapy approach. The intervention is predicated on cognitive-based treatment that teaches participants to recognize and examine their negative thoughts, beliefs, and feelings to reprogram their thoughts and gain clearer insight into their problems. This treatment can help relieve distress by stopping the self-blame, shame, and guilt, enabling participants to cope more effectively with life's challenges (Alford & Beck, 1997).

The CYC group intervention consists of 10 weekly 90-minute sessions. Structured and didactic methods based on Women of Color's psychological, social, and political needs and experiences are integrated into each session. These methods include (a) attention to ethnic and gender homogeneity; (b) the use of ethnic matching among participants and facilitator; (c) a focus on themes related to Women of Color's social and psychological development; (d) a termination ritual at the end of the 10-week intervention; and (e) the use of literary works from Black literature to illustrate concepts. This approach is consistent with recent strategies to reduce stress-related symptoms (Miranda et al., 2003; Napholz, 2005) and promote optimal psychosocial functioning (for example, locus of control and coping) among Women of Color (Belgrave et al., 2000; L. V. Jones, 2004, 2009). Although participants are not required to attend a designated number of sessions, they are encouraged to do so because the importance of group cohesion and support is stressed during the orientation after the pretest.

Curriculum Content

Each session consists of a combination of didactic material, literary works, and exercises. For the curriculum to be most effective, the group leader should be familiar with group process, psychosocial competence, and adult development, specifically from a Black feminist perspective and in relation to Women of Color. Given these skill requirements, it is recommended that the group leader be a culturally competent health provider trained in group counseling.

The material for each session is organized around the following headings:

- Goal
- Objectives
- Session rationale
- Technique of engagement
- Materials needed
- Process summary

The protocol includes psychoeducational, social support, and problem-solving approaches to psychosocial competence enhancement. The sessions move from a highly predetermined structure focusing on assigned readings to a progressively more open format. The curriculum covers the following topics.

Overview of Group Program. Weekly sessions can be organized by similar themes and topics that address the goals of the group.

- Session 1: Introduction to the Group Program
- Session 2: Healthy, I Am
- Session 3: The Truth Within
- Session 4: Reconstructing the Self
- Session 5: Life After Stress
- Session 6: Self-Recovery
- Session 7: "The Greatest of These Is Love"
- Session 8: Community
- Session 9: Reconciliation of the Soul
- Session 10: Wrapping Up: A Connection Through Spirit

Group Composition

Ethnic and Gender Homogeneity. The group's ethnic and gender homogeneity (Women of Color) provides an opportunity for more immediate trust and cultural understanding, which can, in turn, foster and enhance group cohesion and deeper self-disclosure (Bernardez, 1983; L. Davis, 1984). This may also lower group conflict, enhance mutual support, and improve attendance, and it may also bring more immediate symptom relief (Johnson & Johnson, 1994; Merta, 1995; Unger, 1989).

Member Selection. The optimal group size is eight to 10 members, which is small enough to create an intimate, sharing environment but large enough to ensure diversity of perspectives and experience. Moreover, this size helps to keep the group cohesive when absences occur (Garvin, 1997; Yalom, 2005). Best practices require a screening and interview with each woman to assess whether she is the right fit for the group's purpose and to balance qualities of other members, including interests, motivation level, and capacity for verbal communication, listening, and sharing. Prospective participants who are excessively dependent, narcissistic, or hostile are not appropriate for this type of group. These vulnerabilities generate poor communication and create relationship difficulties within the group, limiting group participation, process, and progress.

Establishing Norms. The process of establishing rules and clarifying expectations also helps members to identify mutual needs. During the initial session, the group is asked to establish group rules. The most common rules that are agreed on by group members are as follows:

- Respect oneself and one another.
- Agree to disagree.
- What is said in this room stays in this room.
- Attend and be on time.
- Everyone's opinion is valued.

Use of Literature. Both fiction and nonfiction literature authored by Women of Color are used in the group. Group members receive the literature free of charge because asking members to purchase materials may prohibit their participation. Several suggested books are *Mama* by Terry McMillan (1994), *Sisters of the Yam: Black Women and Self-Recovery* by bell hooks (1993), *Family* by J. California Cooper (1991), *Coffee Will Make You Black* by April Sinclair (1994), and *What Looks Like Crazy on an Ordinary Day* by Pearl Cleage (1992). When selecting literature, the group leader should consider the group's reading level and book length; for example, short stories could be great for women with little time to read. The leader must first assess readings for overwhelming and sensitive content such as issues of sexual and physical abuse to determine the extent to which members can cope with this material. Because Women of Color's realities encompass the interaction of multiple variables, including gender, race, ethnicity, class, sexual orientation, religion, and sociopolitical forces, selected books should include several of these variables.

Self-Identification. Consistent with competence development, the use of literary works can facilitate the group process through self-identification with characters in the literature and feedback from group members. When implemented correctly, it can help members face personal challenges. Group members often identify with characters in the readings. Once members identify and discuss themes from the literature, they can discuss how these characters and their problems and routes out of them relate to their personal experiences. Discussion of the readings enables members to receive feedback while also receiving support on issues they face. The readings provide a model of cultural adaptation to sudden, constant, and future change.

Group Process. The 10-session group is structured to meet for 90 minutes weekly. The sessions move from being highly structured, focused on assigned readings, to a progressively more open format. Sessions begin with less intimate content and move toward more intimate topics. This group process enables members to gain insight into their personal and environmental stressors and to acquire new skills such as clear communication of needs, assertiveness, constructive confrontation, and negotiation skills that are associated with positive and strong self-esteem.

Although specific themes are covered each week, the group process is such that themes are woven throughout sessions, and more than one theme can surface at a time. For instance, in discussing the book *Sisters of the Yam*, session 2 of the group program focuses on the link between dedication to honesty with self and the capacity to be healthy through self-care, with an eye toward enhancing participants' self-attitude. This construct of competence is further explored in sessions 4 and 5, in which participants once again examine ways to develop a positive Black, female self-concept.

Curriculum Content. Each of the 10 sessions consists of a combination of didactic material, literary works, and exercises. The group leader should be experienced in group processes, psychosocial dynamics, and adult development, specifically in relation to Women of Color. The protocol includes psychoeducational, social support, and problem-solving approaches to enhancing psychosocial competence and alleviating depression symptoms. Table 1 outlines the sessions, the session goals, the desired individual outcomes, and the general interventions.

Group Leadership. It is recommended that the group leader be a Black, female professional woman trained in group work. Fenster (1996) suggested that therapeutic support groups for particular populations may be most effective when adapted to include close ties with professionals and conventional services. Research has indicated that for Black Americans, an ethnic match between the leader and group members is related to longer treatment length, fewer dropouts after one session, and markedly improved outcomes on global evaluation measures (L. V. Jones, 2008; Lopez & Lopez, 1993). In addition, facilitators who are the same race and gender as the members increase the likelihood that the women will identify with the common experiences, honesty, directness, candor, and openness of the group leaders. In the group intervention model described here, the group leader's role is to structure the group's activities, to see that a safe climate favorable to productive work is maintained, to assist in facilitating interaction, to provide information and feedback aimed at helping members see alternatives to their modes of behavior, and to encourage them to translate their insights into action plans (Lopez & Lopez, 1993).

In addition to representing a beacon for social work practice and for Women of Color, Black feminist therapy can serve as a political movement in combating the numerous complex oppressions and psychosocial stressors faced by Women of Color. Black feminist therapy practice methods help Women of Color improve their self-image by repudiating the constructs of the patriarchal and racist society and rejecting the shame and degradation induced by social and cultural norms. It can also assist in consciousness-raising, which can also help Women of Color better cope with the stressors and problems they face. Hence, the incorporation of Black feminist practice perspectives that raise consciousness, foster resilience, and empower Women of Color will serve to decrease psychosocial stressors and promote positive coping strategies (Boyd-Franklin, 2006; L. V. Jones & Warner, 2011; Vaz, 2005). Moreover, they will assist social workers and other mental health practitioners in cultivating modes of empowerment that Women of Color and practitioners may use to develop positive mental health outcomes. These outcomes can include realization of one's potential, positive coping strategies, improved quality of life, and positive influence on lifestyle and behavior (L. V. Jones, 2015; L. V. Jones & Warner, 2011; Thomas & González-Prendes, 2009).

TABLE 1: Session Modules, Activities, and Outcomes

Module	Session Activities	Target Outcomes
Psychological, social, and cultural effects of oppression	Examine racial and gender oppression. Engage in self-definition exercise. Discuss the role of stress in participants' lives and identify strategies for coping.	Stress reduction Depressive symptoms Coping
Black female identity	Examine historical and current internalized negative self-attitudes using a self-attitudes and truth-telling exercise. Revisit coping strategies and explore traditional familial coping methods. Discuss restrictive and constructive thinking as they relate to coping from a culturally relevant perspective. Acknowledge and affirm the status of being Black and female.	Stress reduction Depressive symptoms Coping Mastery and control
Healthy relationships	Examine love as it relates to self, family, and romantic relationships. Complete exercise on negative and positive love practices. Explore compassion and forgiveness as they relate to healthy relationships and engage in reconciliation exercise.	Stress reduction Depressive symptoms Mastery and control
Social support	Define social support and discuss strategies for a collective healing process. Complete "Creating Our Community" exercise.	Stress reduction Social support

TREATMENT BENEFITS

For participants in this culturally specific group intervention, healing involves the acknowledgment and validation of both their current and historical realities of unrecognized or devalued relationships, denigration of success, and undue destructive criticism of normative difficulties. Group members learn to hear each other's deepest fears, insecurities, and mistakes in the context of informed, nonjudgmental, and caring relationships. They learn to develop self-empathy and compassion for their own vulnerabilities, imperfections, and mistakes. Through this process, members often feel empowered to take control of their life outcomes and to actively cope with difficult life circumstances. Three strategies of this culture-specific group that engender change are (1) exploration of stressors that affect participants' ability to develop competence; (2) sharing and validation of each other's experiences from their shared and unique perspectives; and (3) development of the problem-solving skills necessary to cope with stressors of daily living. This process of change requires that members become engaged in a supportive therapeutic environment in which they can hear, see, acknowledge, and affirm perceptions, needs, values, and experiences.

Evidence of Treatment Success

This group work program has been used in an array of settings (for example, homeless shelters, early intervention programs, colleges and universities, outpatient and inpatient substance abuse and mental health programs) with Women and Girls of Color. Preliminary studies to examine this program's effectiveness have been conducted by L. V. Jones (2000) and L. V. Jones and Hodges (2002). Additional replication studies have been conducted and have yielded promising data regarding the model's utility with clinical populations (see L. V. Jones, 2004). In L. V. Jones (2004), the sample consisted of 60 Black undergraduate college women between the ages of 18 and 24. The participants were recruited from Boston-area colleges and randomly assigned to three intervention and three no-treatment control groups. Each intervention and control group consisted of 10 members. No statistically significant differences were found between the intervention and control groups on age, college class, parents in the home, hours of work, socioeconomic class, and previous counseling experience. In the three intervention groups, 30 participants were exposed to the psychoeducational group intervention program once a week for eight sessions. The three control groups were not exposed to the intervention, and their participation was limited to completion of the pretest and posttest measures.

The findings of this study (L. V. Jones, 2004) indicated that the culturally specific psychoeducational group program decreased perceived stress for participants in the treatment group compared with those in the control group,

$F(56) = 6.45, p < .01$. These results are supported by previous research on the use of group work with Women of Color (Boyd-Franklin, 2006; Hopps & Pinderhughes, 1999), and they suggest that the group intervention program provided a supportive environment in which members felt comfortable discussing their difficulties in relation to their daily life stressors. The group program may have provided both a direct and an indirect buffer to stress, altering the perception of stress and helping to alleviate stress once experienced. Participants in the intervention group brought into the group process personality and behavioral traits that had been developed on the basis of their experiences and socialization into a society that hinders their ability to develop a healthy internal frame of reference and actively cope. Over time, intervention group participants began to change their perceptions of locus of control and active coping style, which warrants an investigation over an extended period of time.

These findings offer some preliminary data on the effectiveness of this culturally specific group intervention with Women of Color and demonstrate that significant psychosocial changes can be generated in a college setting in a relatively short period of time. This study is a starting point for replication and continuation of the development of culturally relevant group intervention models using a similar research protocol.

An indication of the success of the program in treating Women of Color is demonstrated by the CYC's effectiveness in retaining participants in treatment longer than patients in traditional mental health outpatient services. For Women of Color, this factor is associated with improved client outcomes (S. Sue, 1988; S. Sue, Zane, Nagayama Hall, & Berger, 2009). Moreover, the results demonstrate that treating depression has clear advantages both in relieving daily life stressors and in improving participants' ability to function and better cope with daily life challenges. Given the need for effective, culturally congruent practice, my hope is that the findings and methods can be used along empirically supported lines by our colleagues responsible for transforming services for Women of Color faced with depressive symptoms. Although the specific focus here is Women of Color, the ideas presented may be applicable to other groups and thus beneficial in a broader multicultural context.

CHAPTER QUESTIONS

1. In what ways might this group be useful in working with Women of Color?

2. Was it surprising to find that external locus of control and coping had nonsignificant results? Please explain why.

3. What themes or topics might you consider in addition to those listed?

4. What are your thoughts about incorporating literature into therapy with Women of Color?

CHAPTER 8

Conclusion: Black Feminist Therapy, a 21st Century Imperative

Although Communities of Color have often deemed mental illness "the White man's disease," over the past several years we have witnessed Women of Color—namely, celebrities—coming out on television and social media about their mental health struggles and consequent resilience—for example, the iconic Serena Williams revealed that she had postpartum depression, and Mariah Carey, Halle Berry, Eva Longoria, and Salma Hayek all disclosed that they have struggled with depression, anxiety, bipolar disorder, or suicidal thoughts. What we have observed is that mental illness does not discriminate; women of any race, class, sexuality, or disability status can be affected. For a woman who refuses to seek help of any kind, the future is likely to be akin to walking on a narrow, downward slope that can end with the development of severe and persistent mental illness.

A major point of this book is to encourage therapists to reenvision wellness versus illness for Women of Color and engage in radical and transformative mental health practices such as Black feminist therapy. Having the wherewithal to engage outside the boundaries of the practice norm and to embrace therapeutic processes and methods that reflect the psychological and social realities faced by Women of Color is one of the most relevant and radical things a therapist can do (L. V. Jones & Warner, 2011). Hence, at the micro level, Black feminist therapy is used to encourage clients to take charge of their own lives (L. V. Jones & Guy-Sheftall, 2017). I hope that *Reenvisioning Therapy with Women of Color: A Black Feminist Healing Perspective* provides the necessary tools for therapists, clients, and educators to take a bold step in the direction of developing awareness and understanding of Women of Color's unique mental health struggles, needs, and resilience.

In writing a book like this, I think it is important to leave readers (therapists, allied professionals, consumers, educators) with a "so what?"—What must we do to reenvision the boundaries of therapy and ensure culturally relevant, effective therapeutic treatment with Women of Color on the micro, macro, and policy levels, as well as culturally relevant research on this treatment?

SO WHAT? ON THE MICRO LEVEL OF PRACTICE

Today more than ever, mental health therapists, allied professionals, educators, and clients need a resource, such as Black feminist therapy, to assist Women of Color in overcoming mental illnesses that strike at the very core of their souls. As underscored in this book, little inquiry into Black feminist therapy or feminist therapy and Women of Color exists in mental health treatment. Just as feminism has been compelled to develop a more inclusive discourse and acknowledge the full array of diversity among women and the effects of oppression on them, mental health therapy will need to similarly evolve. A Black feminist perspective reflects an integrated analysis of race, gender, sexuality, and class in therapy and offers possibilities for working with Women of Color from a holistic framework. It offers therapists a useful method of providing services from a strengths-based perspective, in contrast to models that privilege the prognostic course and treatment of trauma, stress, and coping among Women of Color.

An important goal of Black feminist therapy is to attend to both individual and societal stressors, especially those influenced and exacerbated by experiences of oppression, in an effort to promote positive mental health outcomes among Women of Color. These goals posit a practical perspective on assisting Women of Color to heal the psychological and social damages of racism, sexism, and other forms of oppression that often obstruct self-actualizing behaviors. Moreover, a Black feminist perspective challenges the prevailing notion that gender is the only salient category of oppression in therapy and insists that experiences of White women cannot be generalized to the development of therapeutic treatment strategies for Women of Color. The challenge in the 21st century is to put Black feminist theory into action in mental health practice.

SO WHAT? ON THE MACRO LEVEL OF PRACTICE

Women of Color's attitudes and responses to mental illness may be highly affected both positively and negatively by their cultural environments, including family and community, especially because there is often a belief in Communities of Color that prioritizing mental health is a sign of weakness and that people must be strong when dealing with adversity (Hastings, Martin, & Jones, 2015). These environments influence the meaning Women of Color assign to their mental health as well as how they understand the cause of their illness and the stigma that surrounds mental illness. In addition, their cultural environments affect the pathways they take to obtain mental health services and how well they respond to different types of treatment. Many of the myths about mental illness in Communities of Color are the result of stigma and a lack of understanding of what mental illness is. During a focus group, a consumer shared,

> So, it would help more to reach out to those who are struggling with depression, and have a little compassion about it. Don't put labels on them, you know. Everybody's got a label. "Oh, she crazy [while motioning with her finger]," "He acting just like a crackhead. Oh that's an addict." You know what I'm saying? Or "She's on welfare, you know," or "She ain't never going to be nobody." We got to stop that. Stop labeling people with mental illness, and people got to stop accepting labels, too.

This lack of clarity can lead Women of Color to feel isolated and misunderstood.

Communities of Color (families, schools, churches, social groups) must acknowledge that it is okay to talk about mental illness and resocialize ourselves to understand that mental illness is not the result of character, personal defaults, or cultural predisposition. When we can identify symptoms of mental illness, we must have a common—that is, community—vocabulary to talk about it at home, at school, and at the beauty or barber shop. By engaging in awareness and education, we demystify mental illness. If we are not able to take care of ourselves, our families, and our communities and find healthy ways to cope, we unknowingly internalize many negative messages, which can lead to damage to our spirits. What I have learned from many years of community work is that we have some serious struggles ahead of us, and a lot of those struggles are internal. Stigma and fear are alive and well, and we must continue to battle these beasts. We must learn how to be effective and demonstrate solidarity with People of Color who have mental illness.

Communities of Color cannot in good conscience continue to engage in stigmatizing behavior and ignore the debilitating effects of mental illness. We must begin to prioritize education and awareness, holding communities accountable for the wellness of all of their members. Awareness of and education about mental illness and the treatment process is critical to reducing barriers to treatment for Women of Color. Means of overcoming these barriers may include public education campaigns; educational presentations at community venues; and open information sessions at local hospitals, mental health clinics, and community-based agencies such as churches.

Black feminist therapists can serve in leadership roles that promote equity and inclusiveness for all citizens. Moreover, social media have enabled greater awareness of oppressive acts, especially against women, all over the world. Hence, feminist therapeutic social work practice now has a much broader scope. An overview of such practice even 10 years into the future will likely reveal connections in theory, practice, and policy among practitioners from every corner of the world. With this change in cultural context, we can contemplate becoming a much more caring, compassionate community, one that is not always looking at the bottom line of who is "strong enough." Treatment for Women of Color that posits inclusivity is where Black feminist therapy can once again offer a progressive set of ideas. Hence, change requires awareness and education with corresponding Black feminist activism (action). The expanded understanding of mental health disparities, coupled with the alignment of data, policy, and practice, can help to move the needle and advance mental health equity.

SO WHAT? ON THE POLICY LEVEL OF PRACTICE

For many therapists engaged in sociopolitical change, activism is the precursor to such change. Therapists from feminist; critical; antiracist; structural; and lesbian, gay, bisexual, transgender, and queer–affirmative perspectives have always aligned with anti-oppressive and social change approaches to mental health (Mmatli, 2008; Wehbi & Straka, 2011). With Black feminists being essential to social and political change, the field of mental health clearly should educate therapists on the oppressive and exploitative nature of many institutions (that is, institutionalized sexism, racism, classism, heteronormativity, and ageism). Similarly, Black feminists involved in activism should reveal the connections between Women of Color's mental well-being and injustices among families, communities, and sociopolitical institutions. Moreover, educators should make available training opportunities across mental health fields that offer a chance for students to practice advocacy and political engagement. Programs can augment their policy classes by providing more courses on social action, connecting students to issue-based advocacy groups, and offering greater access to political field practicum placements. Opportunities could include attending grassroots meetings and city or town council hearings or planning a community meeting (Hoefer, 1999). Although such efforts will not make every student into a full-fledged activist, they will likely lessen the widespread complaint that social work programs too often inadequately prepare students for policy practice and political activism.

It is equally important that students be given an opportunity to have firsthand experience in meeting governmental officials, attending political meetings, knocking on doors, chanting at protests, or doing some grassroots fundraising (Rocha, 2000). Consciousness-raising, self-help networks, and therapy groups are often used in conjunction with grassroots or community organizations to help change policies to one day eliminate the biases women face (Pinderhughes et al., 2017). Finally, the profession as a whole can modify its curriculum by including courses that are specific to Women of Color.

I am encouraged by the way in which the political scene is changing, with a shift from conservative White men as the face and voice of the country to liberal Women of Color, heralding that change is necessary and possible. People began to sense this change in 2018 with the surprise gubernatorial nominations of Democrats Stacey Abrams in Georgia and Christine Hallquist, a transgender woman and former electric company executive, in Vermont. We still remember the amazement of Barack Obama's election in 2008 after 27 years in which the office of president was primarily held by Republicans (Reagan, G.H.W. Bush, G. W. Bush). These indicators of a much more diverse, open and democratic body of legislators herald a fundamental change in the social context that should argue for more Black feminist–oriented policies designed to help those who are vulnerable, marginalized, and oppressed.

The impact of Black feminist therapists is far reaching; they have affected the mental health field in many ways and filled a void in mental health counseling. Black feminists' contributions to the field of mental health treatment are reflected in advances in theory and practice; they have also contributed to social and political activism with respect to issues facing Women of Color, such as poverty, job training, equal opportunity, and education. In the field of mental health, consideration of race, gender, sexual identity, sexuality, class, and cultural responsiveness in the etiology, diagnosis, and treatment of Women of Color has until recently been conspicuously absent. Black feminist ideological and philosophical approaches focus on assisting Women of Color and their communities to overcome the constraints of their socialization patterns through empowerment and consciousness-raising about the ways in which they have been and continue to be oppressed, including subtle and overt racism and myth-based gender roles, and ways in which to achieve self-fulfillment and equality, among others. Black feminist research has also helped mental health professionals develop more effective therapy and outcomes, and it has helped to effect change in the mental health community and the broader society through the transformation of social and political institutions.

The absence of work on these important issues stimulated the conceptualization of a Black feminist blueprint for therapeutic practice (L. V. Jones & Guy-Sheftall, 2017), as described in chapter 4. This blueprint proposes a model of consciousness-raising, empowerment, and social and political change because, as Worell and Remer (2003) argued, "fixing" the woman for functioning in a dysfunctional society is insufficient; instead, the dysfunctional society must be fixed.

Last, the Black feminist lens encourages us to look at the uses of power and powerlessness (Pinderhughes et al., 2017) and how status and power hierarchies deprive Women of Color of respect, freedom, and equality. In valuing Women of Color's experiences, therapists and researchers advance the intersectional study of Women of Color as an important endeavor that requires both traditional and innovative methods of research. Black feminists reject the notion of a totally objective science or practice related to behavior and call on educators, researchers, and practitioners to acknowledge their values and biases (Beauboeuf-Lafontant, 2009).

Integral to the success of Black feminisms in therapy is the mental health profession's full-fledged commitment to creating positive outcomes through its development of treatment protocols, delivery of services, and reaffirmation of its values. This commitment can promote equity and social justice for Women of Color and provide an invaluable framework for practice with and research on treatment of all oppressed groups. Black feminist therapists, together with our clients and communities, must work to reconnect care and justice and, in so doing, create a society in which all have the support and opportunities they need to thrive.

APPENDIX

Terminology

Anxiety is an emotion that results from the body's natural reaction to stressful circumstances. It is characterized by feelings of nervousness, apprehension, and worry. Physiological responses such as increased heart rate and blood pressure, sweating, and trembling may also accompany anxiety. People with an anxiety disorder typically have recurring invasive thoughts, restlessness, and worry, and they may avoid certain social settings.

Black feminism is grounded in ideologies of Black women's struggle for equality along the lines of gender, race, capitalism, oppression, political activism, and consciousness. Black feminism holds that the experience of being a Black woman is more than that of being Black or a woman but must be interpreted through these intersecting identities.

Black feminist therapy is a set of related principles arising from what proponents see as a disparity between the origin of most feminist and Afrocentric psychological theories and the majority of Women of Color and other People of Color who seek therapy. These methods and processes offer more complex conceptualizations of gender and its intersections of difference, and they incorporate a fundamental understanding of Black women's historical, sociocultural, familial, and developmental heterogeneity. This perspective recognizes a different way of seeing Black women's reality from a positive standpoint and helps to forge a greater understanding of their strengths, resilience, and struggles.

Black feminist thought expresses Black women's standpoint through theories developed by female Black intellectuals. Black feminist thought acknowledges that the lived experiences of Black women, academic knowledge, and the resulting mental representations of the world are valuable sources to enhance experiences of empowerment. Black feminist thought consists of theoretical interpretations of Black women's reality by those who experience it. Moreover, it is an interpretive framework devoted to explaining the importance of knowledge in maintaining and changing power imbalances.

Cultural congruence refers to the integration of cultural attitudes, beliefs, and values of racial and ethnic minorities into the intervention and the continuous promotion of skills, practices, and interactions in the therapeutic process.

Depression (also known as major depressive disorder or clinical depression) is a common yet severe mental health disorder. It is characterized by symptoms that affect how a person feels, thinks, and handles daily activities and can significantly impair daily life.

Eating disorder is a serious and often fatal illness that causes severe disturbances in a person's eating behaviors. Obsessions with food, body weight, and shape may also signal an eating disorder. Common eating disorders include bulimia nervosa, anorexia nervosa, and binge-eating disorder.

Empowerment occurs when an individual, family, group, or community acquires power. It assumes a position of powerlessness on the part of the client group. Empowerment has been used to help populations of disenfranchised people rise above situations and to foster strength in individuals who experience feelings of powerlessness. For people who occupy powerless roles in more than one area, empowerment assumes that the role of power and powerlessness is integral to the mental health treatment experiences of Women of Color.

Feminist therapy is a collective approach to psychotherapy that focuses on gender and the specific challenges and stressors that women encounter as a result of bias, stereotyping, oppression, discrimination, and other circumstances that negatively affect their mental health.

Gendered racism refers to a form of oppression that occurs as a result of the intersection of race and gender.

Intersectionality is a method of studying the relationships among biological, social, and cultural categorizations such as race, gender, sexual orientation, class, ability, and other axes of identity and how they interact and create interdependent systems of social inequality. Intersectionality holds that the traditional conceptualizations of oppression in society (for example, racism, sexism, homophobia, and religion- or belief-based discrimination) do not act independently of one another; rather, these forms of oppression are interconnected, creating a system of oppression that reflects these intersections.

Mental illnesses, also referred to as *mental health disorders,* are conditions that affect an individual's mood, thinking, and behavior. Examples include depression, schizophrenia, anxiety, and eating disorders.

Power is when an individual, group, culture, institution, or society possesses control, authority, or influence over others.

Powerlessness is when an individual, group, culture, institution, or society lacks the authority or capacity to act or is without strength or resources.

Psychosocial competence emphasizes positive mental health or adaptive functioning rather than psychopathology. Competence-centered social work practice is conceptualized as a multifaceted configuration that includes a set of self-attitudes and world and behavioral attributes designed to promote effective functioning in human beings by focusing on their unique adaptive and coping patterns, actual or potential strengths, natural helping networks, life experiences, and environmental resources as major instruments of intervention.

Psychosocial stressors result from social interactions and an imbalance between demands placed on individuals and their ability to manage them. Examples of such interactions are pregnancy, imprisonment, divorce, child abuse, bullying, war, illness, poverty, and caring for an ailing parent or disabled child.

Political activism is a doctrine or practice that consists of direct vigorous efforts to promote, impede, or intervene in reform and create awareness about specific political issues.

Radical feminism is a perspective within feminism that calls for a radical rearrangement of society in which male supremacy is eradicated in all social and economic contexts. A central tenet of radical feminism is that women are oppressed globally by men.

Sexual violence is defined as a sexual act committed against someone without that person's freely given consent.

Standpoint refers to experiences that are historically shared within a group. This theoretical perspective argues that knowledge arises from social position. Standpoint theory also argues that groups who share a common position in hierarchical power relations also have collective experiences in such power relations.

The Personal Is Political (also "The Private Is Political") is a feminist political and theoretical slogan that expresses the relationship among the personal experiences of women, sociopolitical structures, and gender inequality.

Wellness is a way of living with a goal of optimal health and well-being through integration of the mind, body, and spirit while maximizing an individual's potential. Through wellness, individuals are able to live a fuller life within the social and natural community.

References

Abrams, J. A., Maxwell, M., Pope, M., & Belgrave, F. Z. (2014). Carrying the world with the grace of a lady and the grit of a warrior: Deepening our understanding of the "strong Black woman" schema. *Psychology of Women Quarterly, 38*, 503–518.

Aiyer, S. M., Zimmerman, M. A., Morrel-Samuels, S., & Reischl, T. M. (2015). From broken windows to busy streets: A community empowerment perspective. *Health Education & Behavior, 42*, 137–147. doi:10.1177/1090198114558590

Alegría, M., Atkins, M., Farmer, E., Slaton, E., & Stelk, W. (2010). One size does not fit all: Taking diversity, culture, and context seriously. *Administration and Policy in Mental Health, 47*(1–2), 48–60.

Alegría, M., Canino, G., Rios, R., Vera, M., Calderón, J., Rusch, D., & Ortega, A. N. (2002). Mental health care for Latinos: Inequalities in use of specialty mental health services among Latinos, African Americans, and non-Latino whites. *Psychiatric Services, 53*, 1547–1555.

Alexander, M. (2010). *The new Jim Crow: Mass incarceration in the age of colorblindness.* New York: New Press.

Alford, B. A., & Beck, A. T. (1997). *The integrative power of cognitive therapy.* New York: Guilford Press.

Alvidrez, J., & Azocar, F. (1999). Distressed women's clinic patients: Preferences for mental health treatments and perceived obstacles. *General Hospital Psychiatry, 21*, 340–347.

American Psychiatric Association. (2013). *Diagnostic and statistical manual of mental disorders* (5th ed.). Arlington, VA: American Psychiatric Publishing.

American Psychological Association. (2019). *Ethnic and racial minorities & socioeconomic status*. Retrieved from https://www.apa.org/pi/ses/resources/publications/minorities

Artinian, N. T., Washington, O. G., Flack, J. M., Hockman, E. M., & Jen, K. L. (2006). Depression, stress and blood pressure in urban African American women. *Progress in Cardiovascular Nursing, 21*(2), 68–75.

Asante, M. K. (1992). *Afrocentricity*. Trenton, NJ: Africa World Press.

Austin, D. M. (2000). Greeting the second century: A forward look from a historical perspective. In J. G. Hopps & R. Morris (Eds.), *Social work at the millennium: Critical reflections on the future of the profession* (pp. 18–41). New York: Free Press.

Baldwin, J. (2010). Black English: A dishonest argument. In R. Kenan (Edl), *The cross of redemption: Uncollected writings* (pp. 154–159). New York: Pantheon Books.

Bales, R. F. (1965). The equilibrium problem in small groups. In A. P. Hare, E. F. Borgatta, & R. F. Bales (Eds.), *Small groups: Studies in social interaction* (pp. 424–456). New York: Knopf.

Barnes, J. S., & Bennett, C. E. (2002). *The Asian population: 2000*. Washington, DC: U.S. Census Bureau.

Beauboeuf-Lafontant, T. (2009). *Behind the mask of the strong Black woman: Voice and the embodiment of a costly performance*. Philadelphia: Temple University Press.

Belgrave, F. Z., Chase-Vaughn, G., Gray, F., Addison, J. D., & Cherry, V. R. (2000). The effectiveness of a culture and gender-specific intervention for increasing resiliency among African American preadolescent females. *Journal of Black Psychology, 26*, 133–147. doi:10.1177/0095798400026002001

Bernardez, T. (1983). Women's groups. In M. Rosenbaum (Ed.), *Handbook of short term therapy groups* (pp. 119–138). New York: McGraw-Hill.

Blazer, D. G., & Hybels, C. F. (2000). Marked differences in antidepressant use by race in an elderly community sample: 1986–1996. *American Journal of Psychiatry, 157*, 1089–1095.

Blazer, D., Hybels, C., Simonsick, E., & Hanlon, J. T. (2000). Sedative, hypnotic, and antianxiety medication use in an aging cohort over ten years: A racial comparison. *Journal of the American Geriatrics Society, 48*, 1073–1079.

Borum, R. (2012). Radicalization into violent extremism II: A review of conceptual models and empirical research. *Journal of Strategic Security, 4*(4), 37–62.

Bowie, S. L., & Dopwell, D. M. (2013). Metastressors as barriers to self-sufficiency among TANF-reliant African American and Latina women. *Affilia, 28*, 177–193.

Bowleg, L., Huang, J., Brooks, K., Black, A., & Burkholder, G. (2003). Triple jeopardy and beyond: Multiple minority stress and resilience among Black lesbians. *Journal of Lesbian Studies, 7*, 87–108.

Boyd-Franklin, N. (1991). Recurrent themes in the treatment of African American women in group therapy. *Women and Therapy, 11*(2), 25–40.

Boyd-Franklin, N. (2006). *Black families in therapy: Understanding the African American experience.* New York: Guilford Press.

Braun-Williams, C. (1999). African American women, Afrocentrism and feminism: Implications for therapy. *Women & Therapy, 22*(4), 1–16.

Brown, C., & Palenchar, D. (2004). Treatment of depression in African American primary care patients. *African American Research Perspectives, 10*, 55–65.

Brown, L. M., & Gilligan, C. (1992). *Meeting at the crossroads: Women's psychology and girls development.* New York: Ballantine Books.

Brown, L. S. (1994). *Subversive dialogues: Theory in feminist therapy.* New York: Basic Books.

Brown, L. S. (2018). *Feminist therapy* (2nd ed.). Washington, DC: American Psychological Association.

Brown, T. L., Linver, M. R., & Evans, M. (2010). The role of gender in the racial and ethnic socialization of African American adolescents. *Youth & Society, 41*, 357–381. https://doi.org/10.1177/0044118X09333665

Brown, T., & Smith, R. A. (2009). *Latino women and gender issues.* New York: Columbia University Libraries.

Browne, C., & Mills, C. (2001). Theoretical frameworks: Ecological model, strengths perspective, and empowerment theory. In R. Fong & S. Furlito (Eds.), *Culturally competent practice: Skills, interventions and evaluations* (pp. 10–32). Boston: Allyn & Bacon.

Bruce, M. A., & Thornton, M. C. (2004). It's my world? Exploring Black and white perceptions of personal control. *Sociological Quarterly, 45*, 597–612.

Bureau of Labor Statistics. (2016). *Labor force characteristics by race and ethnicity, 2015.* Retrieved from https://www.bls.gov/opub/reports/race-and-ethnicity/2015/home.htm

Cade Bambara, T. (1970). *The Black woman: An anthology.* New York: Simon & Schuster.

Cade Bambara, T. (1980). *The salt eaters.* New York: Random House.

Campinha-Bacote, J. (2008). People of African-American heritage. In L. Purnell & B. Paulanka (Eds.), *Transcultural health care: A culturally competent approach* (3rd ed., pp. 56–74). Philadelphia: F. A. Davis.

Carr, E. S. (2003). Rethinking empowerment theory using a feminist lens: The importance of process. *Affilia, 18*(1), 8–20.

Carrington, C. H. (2006). Clinical depression in African American women: Diagnoses, treatment, and research. *Journal of Clinical Psychology, 62*, 779–791.

Choi, N. G., & Gonzalez, J. M. (2005). Geriatric mental health clinicians' perceptions of barriers and contributors to retention of older minorities in treatment: An exploratory study. *Clinical Gerontologist, 28*(3), 3–25.

Clark, R., Anderson, N. B., Clark, V. R., & Williams, D. R. (1999). Racism as a stressor for African Americans: A biopsychosocial model. *American Psychologist, 54*, 805–816.

Cleage, P. (1992). *What looks like crazy on an ordinary day.* New York: Avon.

Collins, P. H. (2000). *Black feminist thought: Knowledge, consciousness, and the politics of empowerment.* New York: Routledge.

Comas-Díaz, L. (2010). Multicultural approaches to psychotherapy. In J. C. Norcross, G. R. VandenBos, & D. K. Freedheim (Eds.), *History of psychotherapy: Continuity and change* (2nd ed., pp. 243–267). Washington, DC: American Psychological Association.

Comas-Díaz, L. (2012). Humanism and multiculturalism: An evolutionary alliance. *Psychotherapy, 49*(4), 437-441.

Comas-Díaz, L. (2014). Feminist therapy with Hispanic/Latina women: Myth or reality? In L. Fulani (Ed.), *The psychopathology of everyday racism and sexism* (pp. 39–61). New York: Psychology Press.

Comas-Díaz, L. (2015). *Multicultural care: A clinician's guide to cultural competence.* Washington, DC: American Psychological Association.

Comas-Díaz, L., & Greene, B. (1994). Overview: Gender and ethnicity in the healing process. In L. Comas-Díaz & B. Greene (Eds.), *Women of color: Integrating ethnic and gender identities in psychotherapy* (pp. 185–193). New York: Guilford Press.

Comas-Díaz, L., & Jacobsen, F. M. (2001). Ethnocultural allodynia. *Journal of Psychotherapy Practice & Research, 10*, 246–252.

Combahee River Collective. (1986). *The Combahee River Collective statement: Black feminist organizing in the seventies and eighties.* Albany, NY: Kitchen Table.

Conner, K. O., Copeland, V. C., Grote, N. K., Rosen, D., Albert, S., McMurray, M. L., et al. (2010). Barriers to treatment and culturally endorsed coping strategies among depressed African-American older adults. *Aging and Mental Health, 14*, 971–983.

Constantine, M. (2002). Racism attitudes, white racial identity attitudes, and multicultural counseling competence in school counselor trainees. *Counselor Education & Supervision, 41*, 162–174.

Cooper, A. J. (1892). *A voice from the south: By a Black woman of the south.* Xenia, OH: Aldine.

Cooper, J. C. (1991). *Family.* New York: Anchor.

Cooper-Patrick, L., Powe, N. R., Jenckes, M. W., Gonzales, J. J., Levine, D. M., & Ford, D. E. (1997). Identification of patient attitudes and preferences regarding treatment of depression. *Journal of General Internal Medicine, 12*, 431–438. doi:10.1046/j.1525-1497.1997.00075.x

Cuijpers, P. (1998). Psychological outreach programmes for the depressed elderly: A meta-analysis of effects and dropout. *International Journal of Geriatric Psychiatry, 13*(1), 41–48.

Cummings, J. R., & Druss, B. G. (2011). Racial and ethnic differences in mental health service use among adolescents with major depression. *Journal of the American Academy of Child & Adolescent Psychiatry, 50*, 160–170.

Dash, J. (2006). I am the utterance of my name. In T. Tsenes-Hill (Ed.), *I am the utterance of my name: Black Victorian feminist discourse and intellectual enterprise at the Columbian Exposition, 1893* (pp. 92–118). New York: iUniverse.

Davis, K. (2005). *Decreasing discrimination and stigma associated with mental illness in the African American community*. Retrieved from www.stopstigma.samhsa.gov/archtel.htm

Davis, L. (1984). Essential components of group work with Black Americans. *Social Work with Groups, 7*(3), 97–109.

Davis, T. A., & Ancis, J. (2012). Look to the relationship: A review of African American women substance users' poor treatment retention and working alliance development. *Substance Use and Misuse, 47*, 662–672.

Dean, R. (2001). The myth of cross cultural competence. *Families in Society, 82*, 623–630.

Delahanty, J., Ranganathan, R., Postrado, L., Balis, T., Green-Paden, L., & Dixon, L. (2001). Differences in rates of depression in schizophrenia by race. *Schizophrenic Bulletin, 27*(1), 29–37.

DeNavas-Walt, C., Proctor, B. D., & Smith, J. (2008). *Income, poverty, and health insurance coverage in the United States: 2007*. Washington, DC: U.S. Census Bureau.

Denton, T. (1990). Bonding and supportive relationships among Black professional women: Rituals of restoration. *Journal of Organizational Behavior, 11*, 447–457.

Dill, B. T., McLaughlin, A., & Nieves, A. D. (2007). Future directions of feminist research: Intersectionality. In S. Hesse-Biber (Ed.), *Handbook of feminist research, theory, and praxis* (pp. 629–638). Thousand Oaks, CA: Sage Publications.

Deutsch, H. (1945). *The psychology of women: A psychoanalytic interpretation* (Vol. 1: Girlhood; Vol. 2: Motherhood). New York: Green and Stratton.

Donovan, R. A., Galban, D. J., Grace, R. K., Bennett, J. K., & Felicié, S. Z. (2012). Impact of racial macro- and microaggressions in Black women's lives: A preliminary analysis. *Journal of Black Psychology, 39*, 185–196.

Donovan, R. A., & West, L. M. (2014). Stress and mental health: Moderating role of the strong Black woman stereotype. *Journal of Black Psychology, 41*, 384–396.

Edge, D., Baker, D., & Rogers, A. (2004). Perinatal depression among Black Caribbean women. *Health and Social Care in the Community, 12*, 430–438.

Ehrmin, J. T. (2005). Dimensions of culture care for substance-dependent African American women. *Journal of Transcultural Nursing, 16*, 117–125.

Enns, C. Z. (1997). *Feminist theories and feminist psychotherapies: Origins, themes, and variations.* Binghamton, NY: Harrington Park Press/Haworth Press.

Espín, O. M. (1993). Feminist therapy: Not for or by White women only. *Counseling Psychologist, 21*(1), 103–108.

Espín, O. M. (1990). Roots uprooted: Autobiographical reflections on the psychological experience of migration. In F. Alegria & J. Rufinelli (Eds.), *Paradise lost or gained: The literature of Hispanic exile* (pp. 151–163). Houston: Arte Público Press.

Eubanks, R. L., McFarland, M. R., Mixer, S. J., Muñoz, C., Pacquiao, D. F., & Wenger, A.F.Z. (2010). Cross cultural communication. *Journal of Transcultural Nursing, 21*(Suppl. 1).

Evans, S. Y., Bell, K., & Burton, N. K. (2017). *Black women's mental health: Balancing strength & vulnerability.* Albany: State University of New York Press.

Evans, D., & Tyler, F. B. (1976). Is work competence enhancing the poor? *American Journal of Community Psychology, 4*, 25–33.

Evans, K. M., Kincade, E. A., Marbley, A. F., & Seem, S. R. (2005). Feminism and feminist therapy: Lessons from the past and hopes for the future. *Journal of Counseling and Development, 83*, 269–277.

Evans, K. M., Seem, S. R., & Kincade, E. A. (2001). A feminist therapist's perspective on Ruth. In G. Corey (Ed.), *Case approach to counseling and psychotherapy* (6th ed., pp. 208–225). Belmont, CA: Wadsworth Brooks/Cole.

Feminist Therapy Institute. (2000). *Feminist Therapy Institute code of ethics (revised, 1999).* Retrieved from http://supp.apa.org/books/Supervision-Essentials/Appendix_D.pdf

Fenster, A. (1996). Group therapy as an effective treatment modality for people of color. *International Journal of Group Psychotherapy, 46*, 399–416.

Flegal, K. M., Carroll, M. D., Ogden, C. L., & Curtin, L. R. (2010). Prevalence and trends in obesity among U.S. adults, 1999–2008. *JAMA, 303*, 235–241.

Ford, C. L., & Airhihenbuwa, C. O. (2010). Critical race theory, race equity, and public health: Toward antiracism praxis. *American Journal of Public Health, 100*(Suppl. 1), S30–S35.

Fortier, J. P., & Bishop, D. (2004). *Setting the agenda for research on cultural competence in health care: Final report.* Rockville, MD: U.S. Department of Health and Human Services, Office of Minority Health.

Freeman, D. (2008). Kenneth B. Clark and the problem of power. *Patterns of Prejudice, 42*(4–5), 413–437.

Fulani, L. (2009). "All power to the people!" In L. Fulani (Ed.), *The psychopathology of everyday racism and sexism* (pp. xi–xix). New York: Psychology Press.

Gardner, J. D., & Enns, C. Z. (2004). Women of Color feminisms and feminist therapy. In J. D. Gardner & C. Z. Enns (Eds.), *Feminist theories and feminist psychotherapies: Origins, themes and variations* (2nd ed., pp. 193–242). New York: Haworth Press.

Garland, J., Jones, H., & Kolodny, R. (1976). A model of stages of group development in social work groups. In S. Bernstein (Ed.), *Explorations in group work* (pp. 17–71). Boston: Charles River.

Garvin, C. D. (1997). *Contemporary group work* (3rd ed.). Boston: Allyn & Bacon.

Garvin, C. D., Gutierrez, L. M., & Galinsky, M. J. (Eds.). (2017). *Handbook of social work with groups*. New York: Guilford Press.

Garza, A. (2014). *A herstory of the #BlackLivesMatter movement by Alicia Garza*. Retrieved from https://thefeministwire.com/2014/10/blacklivesmatter-2/

Gaylord-Harden, N. K., & Cunningham, J. A. (2009). The impact of racial discrimination and coping strategies on internalizing symptoms in African American youth. *Journal of Youth Adolescence, 38*, 532–543.

Geronimus, A. T., Keene, D., Hicken, M., & Bound, J. (2007). Black-white differences in age trajectories of hypertension prevalence among adult women and men, 1999–2002. *Ethnicity and Disease, 17*(1), 40–48.

Giscombe, K. (2018). *Sexual harassment and Women of Color*. Retrieved from http://www.catalyst.org/blog/catalyzing/sexual-harassment-and-women-color

Glass, L. (2012). Help seeking: Perceived risks for African American women. *Affilia, 27*, 95–106.

Glover, T. (2003, December 15). [Review of the book Coming together: Celebrations for African American families, by H. Cole & J. Pinderhughes] *Booklist, 8*, 746–747.

Gnostic Society Library. (n.d.). *The thunder, perfect mind*. Retrieved from http://gnosis.org/naghamm/thunder.html

Goings, K. W. (1994). *Mammy and Uncle Moses: Black collectibles and American stereotyping*. Bloomington: Indiana University Press.

Goldberg, M. (2000). Conflicting principles in multicultural social work. *Families in Society, 81*, 12–21.

Gonzalez, J., Williams, J. W., Noël, P. H., & Lee, S. (2005). Adherence to mental health treatment in a primary care clinic. *Journal of the American Board of Family Practice, 18*(2), 87–96.

Gordon, M. K. (2008). Media contributions to African American girls' focus on beauty and appearance: Exploring the consequences of sexual objectification. *Psychology of Women Quarterly, 32*, 245–256.

Grant, J. G., & Cadell, S (2009). Power, pathological worldviews and the strengths perspective in social work. *Families in Society, 90*, 425–430.

Greene, B. (1994). African American women. In L. Comas-Díaz & B. Greene (Eds.), *Women of Color: Integrating ethnic and gender identities in psychotherapy* (pp. 10–29). New York: Guilford Press.

Greene, B. (1997). Psychotherapy with African American women: Integrating feminist and psychodynamic models. *Smith College Studies in Social Work, 67,* 299–322.

Greene, B. (2000). African American lesbian and bisexual women. *Journal of Social Issues, 56,* 239–249.

Grieco, E. M., & Cassidy, R. C. (2001). *Overview of race and Hispanic origin, 2000.* Washington, DC: U.S. Department of Commerce, Economics and Statistics Administration.

Griffith, D. M., Mason, M., Yonas, M., Eng, E., Jeffries, V., Plihcik, S., & Parks, B. (2007). Dismantling institutional racism: Theory and action. *American Journal of Community Psychology, 39,* 381–392.

Grote, N. K., Bledsoe, S. E., Larkin, J., Lemay, E. P., & Brown, C. (2007). Stress exposure and depression in disadvantaged women: The protective effects of optimism and perceived control. *Social Work Research, 31,* 19–33.

Grote, N. K., Bledsoe, S. E., Wellman, J., & Brown, C. (2007). Depression in African American and white women with low incomes: The role of chronic stress. *Social Work in Public Health, 23*(2–3), 59–88. doi:10.1080/19371910802148511

Gutierrez, L. M. (1990). Working with women of color: An empowerment perspective. *Social Work, 35,* 149–153.

Guy-Sheftall, B. (1986). Remembering Sojourner Truth: On Black feminism. *Catalyst, 1,* 54–57.

Guy-Sheftall, B. (1995). *Words of fire: An anthology of African-American feminist thought.* New York: New Press.

Guy-Sheftall, B. (2005). African-American studies: Legacies & challenges: "What would black studies be if we'd listened to Toni Cade?" *Black Scholar, 35*(2), 22–24. doi:10.1080/00064246.2005.11413308

Guzmán, B. (2001). *The Hispanic population: Census 2000 brief.* U.S. Department of Commerce. Economics and Statistics Administration. U.S. Census Bureau. Retrieved from http://www.census.gov/prod/2001pubs/c2kbr01-3.pdf

Handy, F., & Kassam, M. (2006). Practice what you preach? The role of rural NGOs in women's empowerment. *Journal of Community Practice, 14*(3), 69–91.

Harley, D. A., Jolivette, K., McCormick, K., & Tice, K. (2002). Race, class, and gender: A constellation of positionalities with implications for counseling. *Journal of Multicultural Counseling and Development, 30,* 216–238.

Harrell, S. P. (2000). A multidimensional conceptualization of racism-related stress: Implications for the well-being of people of color. *American Journal of Orthopsychiatry, 70,* 42–57.

Harrington, E. F., Crowther, J. H., & Shipherd, J. C. (2010). Trauma, binge eating, and the "strong Black woman." *Journal of Consulting and Clinical Psychology, 78,* 469–479. doi:10.1037/a0019174

Harris, T. E., & Sherblom, J. C. (2008). *Small group and team communication.* Boston: Pearson.

Hastings, J. F., Martin, P. P., & Jones, L. V. (2015). *African Americans and depression: Signs, awareness, treatments, and interventions.* Lanham, MD: Rowman & Littlefield.

Hernández-Ronquillo, L., Téllez-Zenteno, J. F., Garduño-Espinosa, J., & González-Acevez, E. (2003). Factors associated with therapy noncompliance in type-2 diabetes patients. *Salud pública de México, 45,* 191–197.

Hines-Martin, V., Malone, M., Kim, S., & Brown-Piper, A. (2009). Barriers to mental health care access in an African-American population. *Issues in Mental Health Nursing, 24,* 237–256.

Hoefer, R. (1999). The social work and politics initiative: A model for increasing political content in social work education. *Journal of Community Practice, 6*(3), 71–87.

hooks, b. (1981). *Ain't I a woman: Black women and feminism.* Boston: South End Press.

hooks, b. (1984). *Feminist theory: From margin to center.* Boston: South End Press.

hooks, b. (1993). *Sisters of the yam: Black women and self-recovery.* New York: Routledge.

hooks, b. (2000). *Feminism is for everybody: passionate politics.* Boston: South End Press.

Hopps, J. G., & Pinderhughes, E. B. (1999). *Group work with overwhelmed clients.* New York: Free Press.

Hopps, J. G., Pinderhughes, E. B., & Shankar, R. (1995). *The power to care.* New York: Free Press.

Hoyt, E. H., & Beard, H. (2009). *Health first: The Black women's wellness guide.* New York: Smiley Books.

Husband, C. (2000). Recognizing diversity and developing skills: The proper role of transcultural communication. *European Journal of Social Work, 3,* 225–234.

Institute of Medicine, Committee on Understanding and Eliminating Racial and Ethnic Disparities in Health Care. (2003). *Unequal treatment: Confronting racial and ethnic disparities in health care.* Washington, DC: National Academies Press.

Institute for Women's Policy Research. (2017). *The gender wage gap: 2016 earnings differences by gender, race, and ethnicity.* Retrieved from https://iwpr.org/publications/gender-wage-gap-2016-earnings-differences-gender-race-ethnicity/

Jackson, J., Neighbors, H. W., Torres, M., Martin, L. A., Williams, D. R., & Blaser, R. (2007). Use of mental health services and subjective satisfaction with treatment among Black Caribbean immigrants: Results from the National Survey of American Life. *American Journal of Public Health, 97,* 60–67.

Jackson, L. C., & Greene, B. (2000). *Psychotherapy with African American women: Innovations in psychodynamic perspectives and practice.* New York: Guilford Press.

Jackson, V. (2017). Power-based therapy: Transforming powerlessness into power. In E. Pinderhughes, V. Jackson, & P. Romney (Eds.), *Understanding power: An imperative for human services* (pp. 55–70). Washington, DC: NASW Press.

Jarama, S. L., Belgrave, F., & Zea, M. C. (1996). The role of social support in adaptation to college among Latino students. *Cultural Diversity and Mental Health, 2,* 193–203.

Jenkins, Y. M. (1993). African-American women: Ethnocultural variables and dissonant expectations. In J. L. Chin, V. De La Cancela, & Y. M. Jenkins (Eds.), *Diversity in psychotherapy: The politics of race, ethnicity and gender* (pp. 117–135). Westport, CT: Praeger.

Johnson, D. W., & Johnson, F. P. (1994) *Joining together: Group theory and group skills* (5th ed.). Boston: Allyn & Bacon.

Jones, A. (Ed.), Eubanks, V. (Ed.), & Smith, B. (2014). *Ain't gonna let nobody turn me around: Forty years of movement building with Barbara Smith.* Albany: State University of New York Press.

Jones, C. (2002). Confronting institutionalized racism. *Phylon, 50,* 7–22.

Jones, L. V. (2000). *Enhancing psychosocial competence among Black women through an innovative psycho-educational group intervention.* Ann Arbor, MI: UMI Publishing/Bell & Howell.

Jones, L. V. (2004). Enhancing psychosocial competence among Black women in college. *Social Work, 49,* 75–84.

Jones, L. V. (2008). Preventing depression: Culturally relevant group work with Black women. *Journal of Research on Social Work Practice, 18,* 626–634. doi:10.1177/1049731507308982

Jones, L. V. (2009). Claiming your connections: A psychological group intervention study of Black college women. *Social Work Research, 33,* 159–171. doi:10.1093/swr/33.3.159

Jones, L. V. (2015). Black feminisms: Renewing sacred healing spaces. *Affilia, 30,* 246–252. doi:10.1177/0886109914551356

Jones, L. V. (2017). The power to recover: Psychosocial competence interventions with Black women. In E. Pinderhughes, V. Jackson, & P. A. Romney (Eds.), *Understanding power: An imperative for human services* (pp. 87–100). Washington, DC: NASW Press.

Jones, L. V., Ahn, S., & Chan, K. T. (2014). Expanding the psychological wellness threshold for Black college women: An examination of the Claiming Your Connections intervention. *Research on Social Work Practice, 26*, 399–411. doi:10.1177/1049731514549631

Jones, L. V., Ahn, S., Quezada, N. M., & Chakravarty, S. (2018). Enhancing counseling services for Black college women attending HBCUs. *Journal of Ethnic & Cultural Diversity in Social Work*. doi:10.1080/15313204.2018.1449689

Jones, L. V., & Ford, B. (2008). Depression in African American women: Application of a psychosocial competence practice framework. *Affilia, 23*(2), 134–143.

Jones, L. V., & Guy-Sheftall, B. (2015). Conquering the Black girl blues. *Social Work, 60*, 343–350.

Jones, L. V., & Guy-Sheftall, B. (2017). Black feminist therapy as a wellness tool. In S. Y. Evans, K. Bell, & N. K. Burton (Eds.), *Black women's mental health: Balancing strength and vulnerability* (pp. 201–213). Albany: SUNY Press.

Jones, L. V., & Harris, M. A. (2018). Developing a Black feminist analysis for mental health practice: From theory to praxis. *Women & Therapy, 42*, 251–264.

Jones, L. V., & Hodges, V. (2002). Enhancing psychosocial competence among Black women: A psycho-educational group model approach. *Social Work with Groups, 24*(3–4), 33–52. doi:10.1300/J009v24n03_04

Jones, L. V., & Warner, L. (2011). Evaluating culturally responsive group work with Black women. *Journal of Research on Social Work Practice, 21*, 737–746. doi:10.1177/1049731511411488

Jones, S. J. (2003). Complex subjectivities: Class, ethnicity, and race in women's narratives of upward mobility. *Journal of Social Issues, 59*, 803–820.

Kaslow, F. W., & Magnavita, J. J. (2002). *Comprehensive handbook of psychotherapy, psychodynamic/object relations*. New York: Wiley.

Keating, F., Robertson, D., McCulloch, A. W., & Francis, E. (2002). *Breaking the circles of fear*. London: Sainsbury Centre for Mental Health.

King, D. (1988). Multiple jeopardy, multiple consciousness: The context of a Black feminist ideology. *Journal of Women in Culture and Society, 14*(1), 42–72.

Laird, J. (1998). Theorizing culture: Narrative ideas and practice principles. In M. McGoldrick (Ed.), *Re-visioning family therapy* (pp. 20–36). New York: Guilford Press.

Lawson, E. J., Rodgers-Rose, L. F., & Rajaram, S., (1999). The psychosocial context of Black women's health. *Health Care for Women International, 20,* 279–289.

Lee, J.A.B. (2001). *The empowerment approach to social work practice: Building the beloved community* (2nd ed.). New York: Columbia University Press.

Lee, S., Matejkowski, J., & Han, W. (2017). Racial-ethnic variation in mental health service utilization among people with a major affective disorder and a criminal history. *Community Mental Health Journal, 53,* 8–14.

Lewis, J. A., & Grzanka, P. R. (2016). Applying intersectionality theory to research on perceived racism. In A. N. Alvarez, C.T.H. Liang, & H. A. Neville (Eds.), *The cost of racism for people of color: Contextualizing experiences of discrimination* (pp. 31–54). Washington, DC: American Psychological Association.

Lincoln, K. D., Chatters, L. M., Taylor, R. J., & Jackson, J. S. (2007). Profiles of depressive symptoms among African Americans and Caribbean Blacks. *Social Science & Medicine, 65,* 200–213.

Lopez, S. R., & Lopez, A. A. (1993). Mexican Americans' initial preferences for counselors: Research methodologies or researchers' values? *Journal of Counseling Psychology, 40,* 249–251.

Lorde, A. (1981). The uses of anger. *Women's Studies Quarterly, 9*(3), 7–10.

Lum, D. (2011). *Culturally competent practice: A framework for understanding diverse groups and justice issues.* Belmont, CA: Brooks/Cole Cengage Learning.

Maidman Joshua, J., & DiMenna, D. (2000). *Read two books and let's talk next week: Using bibliotherapy in clinical practice.* New York: Wiley.

Maluccio, A. N., Washitz, S., & Libassi, M. F. (1999). Ecologically oriented, competence centered social work practice. In C. W. LeCroy (Ed.), *Case studies in social work practice* (2nd ed., pp. 31–38). Pacific Grove, CA: Brooks/Cole.

Mann, R., Gibbard, G., & Hartman, J. (1967). *Interpersonal styles and group development.* New York: Wiley.

Matos, A. (2015). Feminist psychology: Researchs, interventions and challenges. In I. Parker (Ed.), *Handbook of critical psychology* (pp. 329–338). New York: Routledge.

Matsukawa, L. A. (2001). Group therapy with multiethnic members. In W. Tseng & J. Streltzer (Eds.), *Culture and psychotherapy* (pp. 234–261). Washington, DC: American Psychiatric Publishing.

Matthews, A. K., & Hughes, T. L. (2001). Mental health service use by African American women: Exploration of subpopulation differences. *Cultural Diversity and Ethnic Minority Psychology, 7,* 75–87.

McCall, L. (2005). The complexity of intersectionality. *Journal of Women in Culture and Society, 30,* 1771–1800.

McCubbin, M. (2001). Pathways to health, illness and well-being: From the perspective of power and control. *Journal of Community and Applied Social Psychology, 11*, 75–81.

McGoldrick, M., Giordano, J., & Pearce, J. K. (Eds.). (2005). *Ethnicity and family therapy* (3rd ed.). New York: Guilford Press.

McGuire, T. G., & Miranda, J. (2008). New evidence regarding racial and ethnic disparities in mental health: Policy implications. *Health Affairs, 27*, 393–403.

McKinnon, J. (2003). *The Black population in the United States: March 2002* (Current Population Reports Series P20-541). Washington, DC: U.S. Census Bureau.

McMillan, T. (1994). *Mama*. New York: Pocket Books.

Meleis, A. I., & Hattar-Pollara, M. (1995). Arab American women: Stereotyped, invisible but powerful. In D. Adams (Ed.), *Health issues for Women of Color: A cultural diversity perspective* (pp. 133–163). Thousand Oaks, CA: Sage Publications.

Melfi, C. A., Croghan, T. W., Hanna, M. P., & Robinson, R. L. (2000). Racial variation in antidepressant treatment in a Medicaid population. *Journal of Clinical Psychiatry, 61*, 16–21. doi:10.4088/JCP.v61n0105

Merta, R. J. (1995). Group work: Multicultural perspectives. In J. G. Ponterotto, J. M. Casas, L. A. Suzuki, & C. A. Alexander (Eds.), *Handbook of multicultural counseling* (pp. 567–585). Thousand Oak, CA: Sage Publications.

Miller, J. B. (1973). *Psychoanalysis and women*. Harmondsworth: Penguin Books.

Miller, J. B. (1976). *Toward a new psychology of women*. Boston: Beacon Press.

Miranda, J., Chung, J. Y., Green, B. L., Krupnick, J., Siddique, J., Revicki, D. A., & Belin, T. (2003). Treating depression in predominantly low-income young minority women: A randomized controlled trial. *JAMA, 290*, 57–65.

Miranda, J., & Cooper, L. A. (2004). Disparities in care for depression among primary care patients. *Journal of General Internal Medicine, 19*, 120–126.

Mmatli, T. (2008). Political activism as a social work strategy in Africa. *International Social Work, 51*, 297–310.

Mullings, L. (2006). Resistance and resilience: The Sojourner syndrome and the social context of reproduction in Central Harlem. In A. J. Schulz & L. Mullings (Eds.), *Gender, race, class, and health* (pp. 345–370). San Francisco: Jossey-Bass.

Nadeem, E., Lange, J. M., & Miranda, J. (2009). Perceived need for care among low-income immigrant and U.S. born Black and Latina women with depression. *Journal of Women's Health, 18*, 369–375.

Napholz, L. (2005) An effectiveness trial to increase psychological well-being and reduce stress among African American blue-collar working women.

In K. V. Oxington (Ed.), *Psychology of stress* (pp. 1–16). Hauppauge, NY: Nova Biomedical Books.

National Association of Social Workers. (2015). *Standards and indicators for cultural competence in social work practice.* Retrieved from https://www.socialworkers.org/LinkClick.aspx?fileticket=PonPTDEBrn4%3D&portalid=0

National Center for Cultural Competence. (2009). *The compelling need for cultural and linguistic competence.* Retrieved from https://nccc.georgetown.edu/foundations/need.php

Neal-Barnett, A. (2003). *Soothe your nerves: The Black woman's guide to understanding and overcoming anxiety, panic, and fear.* New York: Fireside Books.

Neal-Barnett, A. M., & Crowther, J. H. (2000). To be female, middle class, anxious, and Black. *Psychology of Women Quarterly, 24,* 129–136.

Neighbors, H. W., Caldwell, C., Williams, D. R., Nesse, R., Taylor, R. J., Bullard, K. M., et al. (2007). Race, ethnicity, and the use of services for mental disorders: Results from the National Survey of American Life. *Archives of General Psychiatry, 64,* 485–494.

Neufeldt, V. (Ed.), & Guralnik, D. B. (Ed.-in Chief Emeritus). (1999). *Webster's new world dictionary of American English* (10th college ed.). New York: Simon & Schuster.

New Freedom Commission on Mental Health. (2003). *Achieving the promise: Transforming mental health care in America. Executive summary* (DHHS Publication No. SMA-03-3831). Rockville, MD: U.S. Government Printing Office.

Nicolaidis, C., Timmons, V., Thomas, M. J., Waters, A. S., Wahab, S., Mejia, A., & Mitchell, S. R. (2010). "You don't go tell white people nothing": African American women's perspectives on the influence of violence and race on depression and depression care. *American Journal of Public Health, 100,* 1470–1476. doi:10.2105/ ajph.2009.161950

Nobles, W. W. (1991). African philosophy: Foundation for Black psychology. In R. L. Jones (Ed.). *Black psychology* (pp. 47–63). Berkeley, CA: Cobb & Henry.

Nugent, F. A., & Jones, K. D. (2009). *Introduction to the profession of counseling.* Upper Saddle River, NJ: Pearson Education.

Nuru-Jeter, A., Dominguez, T. P., Hammond, W. P., Leu, J., Skaff, M., Egerter, S., et al. (2009). "It's the skin you're in": African-American women talk about their experiences of racism. An exploratory study to develop measures of racism for birth outcomes studies. *Maternal Child Health Journal, 13*(1), 29–39.

Office of Research on Women's Health. (2014). *Women of Color health data book* (4th ed.). Bethesda, MD: National Institutes of Health. Retrieved from: https://orwh.od.nih.gov/sites/orwh/files/docs/WoC-Databook-FINAL.pdf

Okazawa-Rey, M., Robinson, T., & Ward, J. V. (1987). Black women and the politics of skin color and hair. *Women & Therapy, 6*(1–2), 89–102. https://doi.org/10.1300/j015v06n01_07

Ono, E. (2013). Violence against racially minoritized women: Implications for social work. *Affilia, 28*, 459–467.

Pack-Brown, S. P., & Fleming, A. (2004). An Afrocentric approach to counseling groups with African Americans. In J. DeLucia-Waack, D. Gerrity, C. Kalodner, & M. T. Riva (Eds.), *Handbook of group counseling and psychotherapy* (pp. 183–199). Thousand Oaks, CA: Sage Publications.

Pinderhughes, E. (1989). *Understanding race, ethnicity, and power: The key to efficacy in clinical practice.* New York: Free Press.

Pinderhughes, E. (2017). Conceptualization of how power operates in human functioning. In E. Pinderhughes, V. Jackson, & P. A. Romney (Eds.), *Understanding power: An imperative for human services* (pp. 1–23). Washington, DC: NASW Press.

Pinderhughes, E., Jackson, V., & Romney, P. (Eds.). (2017). *Understanding power: An imperative for human services.* Washington, DC: NASW Press.

Pistole, M. C. (2004). Editor's note on multicultural competencies. *Journal of Mental Health Counseling, 26*(1), 39–40.

Pollack, S. (2003). Focus-group methodology in research with incarcerated women: Race, power, and collective experience. *Affilia, 18*, 461–472.

Prilleltensky, I., Nelson, G., & Peirson, L. (2001). The role of power and control in children's lives: An ecological analysis of pathways toward wellness, resilience and problems. *Journal Community and Applied Social Psychology, 11*, 143–158.

Proctor, G. (2008). CBT: The obscuring of power in the name of science. *European Journal of Psychotherapy and Counselling, 10*, 231–145.

Quinlan, O. (2012). *Praxis: Bringing theory and practice to teaching.* Retrieved from http://www.oliverquinlan.com/blog/2012/10/23/praxis/#:~:targetText=A%20teacher%20immersed%20in%20praxis,learning%20their%20students%20are%20undertaking.&targetText=Teaching%20is%20a%20complex%20business%20of%20both%20practical%20action%20and%20intellectual%20consideration

Raelin, J. A. (2007). The return of practice to higher education: Resolution of a paradox. *Journal of Higher Education, 56*, 57–77. doi:10.1353/jge.2007.0014

Reid, P. T. (1988). Racism and sexism: Comparisons and conflicts. In P. A. Katz & D. Taylor (Eds.), *Eliminating racism: Profiles in controversy* (pp. 203–221). New York: Plenum Press.

Riordan, R. J., & Wilson, L. S. (1989). Bibliotherapy: Does it work? *Journal of Counseling & Development, 67*, 506–508.

Roberts, A., Jackson, M. S., & Carlton-LaNey, I. (2000). Revisiting the need for feminism and Afrocentric theory when treating African-American female substance abusers. *Journal of Drug Issues, 30*, 901–918.

Rocha, C. J. (2000). Evaluating experiential teaching methods in a policy practice course: The case for service learning to increase political participation. *Journal of Social Work Education, 33*, 433–444.

Romero, R. E. (2000). The icon of the strong Black woman: The paradox of strength. In L. C. Jackson & B. Greene (Eds.), *Psychotherapy with African American women: Innovations in psychodynamic perspectives and practice* (pp. 225–238). New York: Guilford Press.

Rosenthal, S., & Schreiner, A. C. (2000). Prevalence of psychological symptoms among undergraduate students in an ethnically diverse urban public college. *Journal of American College Health, 49*, 12–18.

Russell, D. E., Schurman, R. A., & Trocki, K. (1986). Long-term effects of incestuous abuse in childhood. *American Journal of Psychiatry, 143*, 1293–1296. doi:10.1176/ajp/.143.10.1293

Ryan, R. M., & Deci, E. L. (2000). Self-determination theory and the facilitation of intrinsic motivation, social development, and well-being. *American Psychologist, 55*, 68–78.

Schreiber, R., Stern, P. N., & Wilson, C. (1998). The contexts for managing depression and its stigma among Black West Indian Canadian women. *Journal of Advanced Nursing, 27*, 510–517.

Schulz, A. J., & Mullings, L. (2006). *Gender, race, class, and health: Intersectional approaches.* San Francisco: Jossey-Bass.

Sharf, R. (2003). *Theories of psychotherapy and counseling: Concepts and cases* (3rd ed.). Belmont, CA: Brooks/Cole.

Shechtman, Z. (2000). Bibliotherapy: An indirect approach to treatment of childhood aggression. *Child Psychiatry and Human Development, 30*, 39–53.

Shonfeld-Ringel, S. (2000). Dimensions of cross cultural treatment with late adolescent college students. *Child and Adolescent Social Work Journal, 17*, 443–454.

Short, E. L., & Williams, W. S. (2014). From the inside out: Group work with Women of Color. *Journal for Specialists in Group Work, 39*, 71–91. doi:10.1080/01933922.2013.859191

Sinclair, A. (1994). *Coffee will make you Black: A novel.* New York: HarperCollins.

Smith, B. (Ed.). (1983). *Home girls: A Black feminist anthology.* New York: Kitchen Table.

Snowden, L. R. (1999). African American service use for mental health problems. *Journal of Community Psychology, 27*, 303–313.

Snowden, L. R. (2001). Barriers to effective mental health services for African Americans. *Mental Health Services Research, 3*, 181–187.

Sojourner's Speech. (1851, June 21). Transcribed by Marius Robinson. *Anti-Slavery Bugle* (New-Lisbon, Ohio). Chronicling America: Historic American Newspapers, Library of Congress.

Sommers-Flanagan J. & Sommers-Flanagan R. (2004). *Counseling and psychotherapy theories in context and practice, skills, strategies and techniques.* New Jersey: John Wiley & Sons.

Sparks, E. E., & Parker, A. H. (2000). The integration of feminism and multiculturalism: Ethical dilemmas at the border. In M. M. Brabeck (Ed.), *Practicing feminist ethics in psychology* (pp. 203–224). Washington, DC: American Psychological Association.

Speight, S. L. (2007). Internalized racism: One more piece of the puzzle. *Counseling Psychologist, 35,* 126–134.

Staggenborg, S., & Taylor, V. (2005). Whatever happened to the women's movement? *Mobilization, 10,* 37–52.

Stephens, D. P., & Few, A. L. (2007). The effects of images of African American women in hip hop on early adolescents' attitudes toward physical attractiveness and interpersonal relationships. *Sex Roles, 56*(3–4), 251–264.

Stone, P. T. (1979). Feminist consciousness and Black women. In J. Freeman (Ed.), *Women: A feminist perspective* (pp. 577–588). California City, CA: Mayfield Publishing.

Substance Abuse and Mental Health Services Administration. (2012). *Results from the 2011 National Survey on Drug Use and Health: Mental health findings.* Retrieved from https://www.samhsa.gov/data/sites/default/files/2011MHFDT/2k11MHFR/Web/NSDUHmhfr2011.htm

Sue, D. W., Capodilupo, C. M., & Holder, A. (2008). Racial microaggressions in the life experience of Black Americans. *Professional Psychology: Research and Practice, 39,* 329–336.

Sue, D. W., Capodilupo, C. M., Torino, G. C., Bucceri, J. M., Holder, A.M.B., Nadal, K. L., & Esquilin, M. (2007). Racial microaggressions in everyday life. *American Psychologist, 62,* 271–286.

Sue, D. W., & Sue, D. (2013). *Counseling the culturally diverse: Theory and practice* (4th ed.). New York: Wiley.

Sue, S. (1988). Psychotherapeutic services for ethnic minorities: Two decades of research findings. *American Psychologist, 43,* 301–308.

Sue, S., Zane, N., Nagayama Hall, G. C., & Berger, L. K. (2009). The case for cultural competency in psychotherapeutic interventions. *Annual Review of Psychology, 60,* 525–548. doi:10.1146/annurev.psych.60.110707.163651

Symington, A. (2004, August). *Intersectionality: A tool for gender and economic justice* (AWID Facts & Issues No. 9). Retrieved from https://www.awid.org/publications/intersectionality-tool-gender-and-economic-justice

Taylor, J. Y. (1998). Womanism: A methodologic framework for African American women. *Advances in Nursing Science, 21*(1), 53–61.

Tew, J. (2006). Understanding power and powerlessness: Towards a framework for emancipator practice in social work. *Journal of Social Work, 6,* 33–51.

Thomas, A. J., Witherspoon, K. M., & Speight, S. L. (2008). Gendered racism, psychological distress, and coping styles of African American women. *Cultural Diversity and Ethnic Minority Psychology, 14*, 307–314.

Thomas, S. A., & González-Prendes, A. A. (2009). Powerlessness, anger, and stress in African American women: Implications for physical and emotional health. *Health Care for Women International, 30*(1–2), 93–113.

Thompson, B. W. (1992). "A way outa no way": Eating problems among African-American, Latina, and white women. *Gender & Society, 6*, 546–561. https://doi.org/10.1177/089124392006004002

Thompson, C., & Green, M. R. (1964). *Interpersonal psychoanalysis; the selected papers of Clara M. Thompson, ed. by Maurice R. Green.* New York: Basic Books.

Thompson, C. E., Worthington, R., & Atkinson, D. R. (1994). Counselor content orientation, counselor race, and Black women's cultural mistrust and self-disclosures. *Journal of Counseling Psychology, 41*, 155–161. doi:10.1037//0022-0167.41.2.155

Toseland, R., Jones, L. V., & Gellis, Z. D. (2004). Group dynamics. In C. D. Garvin, L. M. Gutierrez, & M. J. Galinsky (Eds.), *Handbook of social work with groups* (pp. 13–31). New York: Guilford Press.

Toseland, R. W., & Rivas, R. F. (2017). *An introduction to group work practice* (8th ed.). Boston: Pearson.

Truth, S. (1972). What time of night it is. In M. Schneir (Ed.), *Feminism: The essential historical writings* (pp. 96–98). New York: Random House. (Original speech 1853)

Tuckman, B. W. (1965). Developmental sequence in small groups. *Psychological Bulletin, 63*, 384–399. doi:10.1037/h0022100

Tuckman, B. W., & Jensen, M.A.C. (1977). Stages of small-group development revisited. *Group & Organization Studies, 2*, 419–427. doi:10.1177/105960117700200404

Turner, P. A. (1994). *Ceramic uncles and celluloid mammies: Black images and their influence on culture.* New York: Anchor Books.

Tyler, F. B. (1978). Individual psychosocial competence: A personality configuration. *Educational and Psychological Measurement, 38*, 309–323.

Tyler, F. B. (2002). Transcultural ethnic validity model and intracultural competence. In W. J. Lonner, D. L. Dinnel, S. A. Hayes, & D. N. Sattler (Eds.), *Online readings in psychology and culture* (Unit 16, chapter 1). Retrieved from https://scholarworks.gvsu.edu/cgi/viewcontent.cgi?article=1106&context=orpc

Tyler, F. B., Brome, D. R., & Williams, J. E. (1991). *Ethnic validity and psychotherapy: A psychosocial competence approach.* New York: Plenum Press.

Tyler, F. B., & Sinha, Y. (1988). Psychosocial competence and belief systems among Hindus. *Genetic, Social, and General Psychology Monographs, 114*, 33–49.

Unger, R. (1989). Selection and composition criteria in group psychotherapy. *Journal for Specialists in Group Work, 14,* 151–157.

U.S. Census Bureau. (2010). *Selected characteristics of the native and foreign-born populations: 2006-2010 American Community Survey 5-year estimates* [Data file] (American FactFinder version). Retrieved from https://factfinder.census.gov/faces/tableservices/jsf/pages/product view.xhtml?pid=ACS_10_5YR_S0501&prodType=table

U.S. Census Bureau. (2015). *Projections of the size and composition of the U.S. population: 2014 to 2060.* Retrieved from https://www.census.gov/content/dam/Census/library/publications/2015/demo/p25-1143

U.S. Department of Health and Human Services. (2001). *Mental health: Culture, race, and ethnicity: A supplement to mental health: A report to the surgeon general.* Washington, DC: Author.

Utsey, S. O., Ponterotto, J. G., Reynolds, A. L., & Cancelli, A. A. (2000). Racial discrimination, coping, life satisfaction, and self-esteem among African Americans. *Journal of Counseling & Development, 78,* 72–80.

Vaz, K. M. (2005). Reflecting team group therapy and its congruence with feminist principles. *Women & Therapy, 28,* 65–75.

Wade, L. (2011). Sociological images: Loretta Ross on the phrase "Women of Color." Retrieved from https://thesocietypages.org/socimages/2011/03/26/loreta-ross-on-the-phrase-women-of-color/

Waldegrave, C., Tamasese, K., Tuhaka, F., & Campbell, W. (2003). *Just therapy—A journey: A collection of papers from the Just Therapy team, New Zealand.* Adelaide, South Australia, Australia: Dulwich Centre Publications.

Wallen, J. (1992). Providing culturally appropriate mental health services for minorities. *Journal of Mental Health Administration, 19,* 288–295.

Wehbi, S., & Straka, S. (2011). Revaluing student knowledge through reflective practice on involvement in social justice. *Social Work Education, 30,* 45–54.

Weiner, G. (1994). *Feminisms in education: An introduction.* Milton Keynes, England: University Press.

Weiss, S. R., Kung, H. C., & Pearson, J. L. (2003). Emerging issues in gender and ethnic differences in substance abuse and treatment. *Current Women's Health Report, 3,* 245–253.

Whaley, A., & Davis, K. (2007). Cultural competence and evidence-based practice in mental health services: A complementary perspective. *American Psychologist, 62,* 563–574.

Whiteford, H. A., Degenhardt, L., Rehm, J., Baxter, A. J., Ferrari, A. J., Erskine, H. E., et al. (2013). The global burden of mental and substance use disorders. *Lancet, 382,* 1575–1586. doi:10.1016/S0140-6736(13)61611-6

Williams, C. B. (2000). African American women, Afrocentrism and feminism: Implications for therapy. *Women & Therapy, 22*(4), 1–16.

Williams, C. B. (2005). Counseling African American women: Multiple identities—multiple constraints. *Journal of Counseling & Development, 83*, 278–283.

Williams, D. R. (2000). Racism and mental health: The African American experience. *Race and Ethnicity, 5*, 243–268.

Williams, D. R., González, H. M., Neighbors, H., Nesse, R., Abelson, J. M., Sweetman, J., & Jackson, J. S. (2007). Prevalence and distribution of major depressive disorder in African Americans, Caribbean Blacks, and non-Hispanic Whites: Results from the National Survey of American Life. *Archives of General Psychiatry, 64*, 305–315.

Wingo, L. K. (2001). Substance abuse in African American women. *Journal of Cultural Diversity, 8*(1), 21–25.

Woods-Giscombé, C. L. (2010). Superwoman schema: African American women's views on stress, strength, and health. *Qualitative Health Research, 20*, 668–683.

Woods-Giscombé, C. L., & Lobel, M. (2008). Race and gender matter: A multidimensional approach to conceptualizing and measuring stress in African American women. *Cultural Diversity and Ethnic Minority Psychology, 14*, 173–182.

Worell, J., & Remer, P. (2003). *Feminist perspectives in therapy: Empowering diverse women* (2nd ed.). Hoboken, NJ: Wiley.

Worell, J., Remer, P., & Worell, J. (1992). *Feminist perspectives in therapy: An empowerment model for women.* Chichester: Wiley.

World Health Organization. (2000). *General guidelines for methodologies on research and evaluation of traditional medicine.* Retrieved from https://apps.who.int/medicinedocs/en/d/Jwhozip42e/

World Health Organization. (2003). *What is the WHO definition of health?* Retrieved from https://www.who.int/about/who-we-are/frequently-asked-questions

Wyatt, G. E. (1992). The sociocultural context of African American and white American women's rape. *Journal of Social Issues, 48*(1), 77–91. https://doi.org/10.1111/j.1540-4560.1992.tb01158

Yalom, I. (2005). *The theory and practice of group psychotherapy* (5th ed.). New York: Basic Books.

Yee, S. J. (1992). *Black women abolitionists: A study in activism, 1828–1860.* Knoxville: University of Tennessee Press.

Zea, M. C., Reisen, C. A., Beil, C., & Caplan, R. D. (1997). Predicting intention to remain in college among ethnic minority and non-minority students. *Journal of Social Psychology, 137*, 149–160.

Zinn, M. B., & Dill, B. T. (1996). Theorizing difference from multiracial feminism. *Feminist Studies, 22*(2), 321–331.

Index

In this index, *t* denotes table.

A

abolitionist movement, 5
Abrams, Stacey, 117
accessibility, 29
acculturation, 14
activism, 61–63, 65, 116, 119
adjourning, in group work, 102–103
alcohol, 38, 59, 68, 83–84
Alexander, Michelle, 59
anxiety, 18, 32, 74, 85–88, 119
assessment
    cultural, 33, 48, 49–50
    internalization and, 75
    race–gender role analysis in, 35
    responsive, 48
    sensitivity in, 33
    sexual victimization and, 75

B

Bambara, Toni Cade, 8, 67
barriers to treatment, 19–20, 29, 30, 33–34, 115
Beale, Francis, 6
beauty, 70–71, 75
bibliotherapy, 100–101, 108
Black feminism, 26, 96, 98–99, 118, 119
Black Feminist Movement, 6, 23, 34
Black feminist therapy, 9–10, 26–37, 40, 52–53, 67–68, 81, 109, 113–118, 119
Black feminist thought, 4–8, 27, 120
Black Feminist Thought: Knowledge, Consciousness, and the Politics of Empowerment (Collins), 8
Black Liberation Movement, 6
Black Lives Matter (BLM), 62–63
Black Women's Truth and Reconciliation Commission, 63
BLM. *See* Black Lives Matter (BLM)
Boyd-Franklin, Nancy, 25–26
BREATHE model, 1

143

Brown, Lyn Mikel, 25
Burke, Tarana, 1

C
capitalization, 3
case studies, 37–38, 50–52, 81–93
Claiming Your Connections (CYC), 95–112, 110t
Clarke, Cheryl, 6
classism, 7, 26, 34, 56, 70, 99, 116
Collins, Patricia Hill, 6, 8, 56
Comas-Díaz, Lillian, 25–26, 31
Combahee River Collective (CRC), 7–8, 62
competence
  cultural, 48, 85
  development, 108, 111
  psychosocial, 10, 61, 64, 95, 96–98, 100, 106, 109, 121
consciousness-raising, 34, 62, 68, 74, 82–85, 86–88, 89–90, 109, 117
Cooper, Anna Julia, 5, 8
cost, of treatment, 29–30
Cullors, Patrisse, 63
cultural assessment, 33, 48, 49–50
cultural barriers, 29, 30
cultural competence, 48, 85
cultural congruence, 95, 120
cultural knowledge building, 49
culturally responsive services, 9, 29, 45–47, 50–52, 64
culture
  defined, 47–50
  group work and, 100, 104–105
CYC. *See* Claiming Your Connections (CYC)

D
Dean, Ruth, 46
depression, 59, 72, 76, 86, 99, 101, 120
Deutsch, Helene, 25
devaluation, 72–74, 99

diagnosis. *See also* misdiagnosis; *specific diagnoses*
  acceptance of, 76
  sensitivity in, 33
diet, 38
Dill, Thornton, 56
disempowerment, 55, 105
diversity
  in group work, 104–105, 107
  and valuation of experience, 31
double victimization, 36, 61
drug abuse, 14–15, 38, 68, 84. *See also* substance abuse

E
eating disorder, 14, 30, 68, 74, 120
ecological perspective, 20, 97
empowerment, 36, 60–61, 64, 82–85, 89–90, 96, 117, 120
Enns, Carol Zerbe, 25
Espín, Olivia, 25
ethnic homogeneity, in group work, 107

F
feminism. *See* Black feminism; radical feminism
feminist psychology, 24, 25, 98
feminist therapy, 24–25, 120. *See also* Black feminist therapy
feminist thought, Black, 4–8
forming, in group work, 102
Frazier, Demita, 62
Freud, Anna, 24

G
Garza, Alicia, 63
gendered racism, 35, 120
Gilligan, Carol, 25
Greene, Beverly, 25–26
group culture, 104–105
group work, 99–109
Guy-Sheftall, Beverly, 5, 6, 7

H

Hallquist, Christine, 117
healing strategies, 34–37
health insurance coverage, 14, 19, 29–30
Henson, Taraji P., 17
hooks, bell, 6, 56
Horney, Karen, 24
hypersensitivity, 72
hypervigilance, 72

I

immigrants, 3, 18, 19, 62
income disparity, 13
internalized oppression, 32–33, 68, 70, 74, 85, 90
internal reflection, 48–49
intersectionality, 20, 27, 56–57, 63, 120
isolation, 56, 64, 70, 84, 100, 105

J

Jackson, Vanessa, 55–56
Jezebel stereotype, 73

K

Keys, Alicia, 17
knowledge building, cultural, 49

L

language, 3, 19, 98
leadership, in group work, 109
literary works, in group work, 100–101, 108
location accessibility, 29
Lorde, Audre, 6, 7, 43

M

machismo, 17
Mahler, Margaret, 24
marianismo, 17
Mendes, Eva, 17

mental health
  defined, 14
  of Women of Color, 17–21
mental health concerns, defined, 14–15
mental health praxis, 23
mental health services utilization
  cultural responsiveness and, 45–47
  minority representation and, 17
  outcomes and, 44–50
mental illnesses, defined, 14, 121
#MeToo, 1, 62, 73
microaggression, 16, 24, 71–72
Milano, Alyssa, 1
Miller, Jean Baker, 25
misdiagnosis, 20, 30, 45, 47, 48
motherhood, 69–70

N

New Jim Crow, The: Mass Incarceration in the Age of Colorblindness (Alexander), 59
Nineteenth Amendment, 5
norming, in group work, 102, 107
nutrition, 38

O

Obama, Barack, 17, 117
online harassment, 16
oppression, 7, 8, 79, 114
  Black feminist thought and, 5
  devaluation and, 73–74
  feminist therapy and, 24
  institutional, 58
  internalized, 29, 32–33, 68, 70, 74, 85, 90
  intersectionality and, 56–57
  power and, 57–60
  simultaneity of, 23
  and Women of Color as term, 4

outcomes
  accessibility and, 29
  health, 18
  mental health services utilization and, 44–50
  power and, 57

P
Parker, Pat, 7
performing, in group work, 102
"The Personal Is Political," 122
personality, powerlessness and, 58–59
political activism, 121. *See also* activism
poverty, 13, 55, 69–70, 117. *See also* classism
power, 55, 57–60, 118, 121
power imbalances, 35–37
powerlessness, 55, 57–60, 118, 121
"power wound," 55–56
praxis. *See* mental health praxis
privilege, 5, 16, 44, 56–59, 69, 82, 114
psychoanalytic theory, 24
psychohistory, 15–17
psychosocial competence, 10, 61, 64, 95, 96–98, 100, 106, 109, 121
psychosocial stressors, 121

R
race–gender analyses, 34–35, 37–38, 92
race–gender–power role process, 39
race–gender role analysis, 35, 86–88, 89–90
race–power gender analysis, 90–93
race–power role analysis, 34, 37–38, 88, 89, 92, 96
racism
  and Black feminist theory, 98, 99
  gendered, 35, 120
  institutional, 59
  and seeking of treatment, 68, 70
  sexism *vs.*, 5
  therapeutic relationship and, 77
  validation of, 53, 78–79
radical feminism, 121
reflection, internal, 48–49
relationship, therapeutic, 24, 31, 37, 40, 52, 60–61, 74–75, 77, 85
relaxation techniques, 39
religion, 30–31, 37, 44, 68, 108
resilience, 32, 70, 84, 98–99, 113
Rodriguez, Gina, 17
Ross, Loretta, 4

S
Salt Eaters, The (Bambara), 67
SBW. *See* "Strong Black Woman" (SBW) mythology
self-esteem, 26, 32, 70–71, 77, 86, 90, 101
self-identification, in group work, 108
self-reflection, 48–49
sensitivity, in assessment and diagnosis, 33, 90–93
sexism
  in Black feminist theory, 98, 99
  racism *vs.*, 5
sexual devaluation, 72–75
sexual victimization, 71, 72–75
sexual violence, 121
slavery, 5, 15, 70, 85
sleep, 39
Sloan, Margaret, 7
Smith, Barbara, 6, 7, 23, 62
Smith, Beverly, 62
spirituality, 30–31. *See also* religion
standpoint, 121–122
stigmatizing behavior, 115
storming, in group work, 102
"Strong Black Woman" (SBW)

mythology, 15–16, 32–33, 75–77
substance abuse, 2, 17, 37, 96, 111. *See also* alcohol; drug abuse
Suffragists, 5

T

therapeutic relationship, 24, 31, 37, 40, 52, 60–61, 74–75, 77, 85
Thompson, Clara, 25
time accessibility, 29
Tometi, Opal, 63
treatment barriers, 19–20, 29, 30, 33–34, 115
Truth, Sojourner, 5

U

utilization, mental health services
    cultural responsiveness and, 45–47
    minority representation and, 17
    outcomes and, 44–50

V

victimhood, inability to admit, 71–72
victimization
    double, 36, 61
    sexual, 71, 72–75

W

Washington, Kerry, 17
wellness, 10, 113, 122
wellness toolbox, 38–39
wellness work, 20
Women of Color
    activism by, 61–63
    college enrollment rates of, 8
    defining, 3–4
    health insurance coverage among, 14
    incidence of mental health disorders among, 2
    income disparity of, 13
    intersectionality and, 56–57
    mental health among, 17–21
    origin of term, 4
    poverty among, 13
    psychohistory of, 15–17
    reasons for seeking treatment, 68–71
    and "Strong Black Woman" mythology, 15–16, 32–33, 74–75
Women's Movement, 6, 24, 62
Worell, Judith, 25, 117

Z

Zinn, Baca, 56

About the Author

Lani V. Jones, PhD, LICSW, is a Black feminist scholar and therapist. She is a professor in the School of Social Welfare and the Department of Women, Gender, and Sexuality Studies at the University at Albany, State University of New York. She has more than 20 years of experience in providing therapy to Women of Color. Her research and scholarship are concentrated in the area of mental health practice research with a focus on enhancing psychosocial competence among Women of Color. Her work includes *African Americans and Depression: Signs, Awareness, Treatments, and Interventions* (Rowman & Littlefield) and numerous articles and book chapters.